A
NEW
BREED
OF
DOCTOR

A NEW BREED OF DOCTOR

ALAN H. NITTLER, M.D.
Foreword by Linda Clark, M.A.

▲
PYRAMID HOUSE
NEW YORK

ISBN 0-515-09313-0

Library of Congress Catalog Card Number: 75-189530

Printed in the United States of America

Pyramid House Books are published by Pyramid Communications, Inc. Its trademarks, consisting of the word "pyramid" and the portrayal of a pyramid, are registered in the United States Patent Office.

PYRAMID HOUSE
Pyramid Communications, Inc.
919 Third Avenue
New York, New York 10022, U.S.A.

Distributed in Canada by Pyramid Books of Canada
888 DuPont Street
Toronto, Canada

CONTENTS

FOREWORD vii
    Linda Clark, M.A.
INTRODUCTION xi

PART I

    I. Thinking Nutritionally 1
   II. Approaches to Treatment 10
 III. My Personal Initiation 27
 IV. Progress—Full Speed Ahead 35
   V. Getting Well Nutritionally 43
 VI. Hypoglycemia: A Common Denominator .. 55
VII. Some Case Histories 65
VIII. Do-It-Yourself Nutrition 87

PART II

    Introduction to Part II 111
 IX. How to Learn Nutritional Know-How.... 113
  X. How I Diagnose and Treat Hypoglycemia.. 128
 XI. Medical Case Histories 152
XII. Nutritional Therapy for the Specialist ... 170
    INDEX 195

Alan H. Nittler, M.D. is "a new breed of doctor" with a new kind of treatment. Why is his treatment different? Because the average doctor is not taught this new science, which we call nutrition, in medical school. Instead the average doctors use drugs which serve as a crutch or to mask the symptoms of disease. The science of nutrition, on the other hand, actually rebuilds the body since the elements which are found in the body by analysis, if fed to the person, help to repair the body or prevent further illness.

Don't take my word for it, or Dr. Nittler's. There are other doctors who are discovering this marvelous, unusual approach to health.

Dr. Nittler is very thorough. He carefully makes exhaustive tests of his new patients to learn what nutrients the patients lack. He also tests for effects of nutritional deficiencies on the body as well as for low blood sugar (called hypoglycemia) because he has found that so many people have this condition and don't know it. When it exists in the patient, it complicates poor health. Fortunately, it can be spotted and controlled and Dr. Nittler is one of the few specialists in the United States who truly understands it.

Dr. Nittler has found that drugs do not produce health—they merely cover up a condition (as aspirin can relieve a headache but not correct the cause). So he helps his patients to rebuild their bodies and actually recover from their disturbances—not merely put up with them. For this reason he does not use a drug except in dire emergencies. I have personally witnessed five lives that he has saved, some of them in an amazingly short time. I have also seen energy and good health return to patients even after years of suffering, unnecessary surgery and hopelessness.

Dr. Nittler has been criticized by those who do not understand his unique approach. Yet he gets most people well, which should be the proof of the pudding. Some of these criticisms have turned into real dillies of distorted rumor, yet his patients, whom he has made well and who know better than those who have not had the treatment, will tell you the truth!

You see, the way Dr. Nittler works, with special emphasis on discovered deficiencies, is that he supplies a smorgasbord of all the elements found by analysis to exist in the body (in the natural form of food, natural vitamins and minerals). The body takes these elements and uses what it needs to repair itself. Many people report that new tissue has, in some cases, replaced the old. Heart sufferers have gone back to work and other ailments too numerous to mention have been brought under control so that the patient can once more lead a comfortable life.

The one question I, as a nutrition reporter and writer, am asked from coast to coast as a result of the three books I have written on the subject is: "Where can I find a nutritional doctor to help me get well?" Unfortunately, I have to write most of these people that there are only a handful of such doctors in existence. To my knowledge there are none in the East or mid-U.S. at all. I always wish, when this question comes in, that I had 5,000 Dr. Nittlers to recommend!

In short, what this country needs is a large supply

of this "New Breed of Doctor."

In this book Dr. Nittler tells how he became one and he tells others how to fulfill the great need of a clamoring public searching for a "new breed of doctor." This book is a breakthrough of courage, help and encouragement. I hope it will be a turning point in awakening everyone, whether patient or doctor, to a realization that the old methods no longer meet the new needs of our present world. A different approach is required to achieve better health and Dr. Nittler explains how it can be put to work in this country. There is no time to lose.

LINDA CLARK, M.A.
*Nutrition Reporter
and Author*

A
NEW
BREED
OF
DOCTOR

INTRODUCTION

*If you wish to know the true value of a physician's
work, do not ask the physician; ask his patients.*

ANON.

THERE IS a medical revolution in the making. Organized medicine as we know it in our society today
is on the ropes. Extreme dogmatism with closed minds
is killing the goose that lays the golden eggs. The
attitude of the organized medical group is that they
know it all, medically speaking, and that no one else
knows anything. Organized medicine is guilty, collectively, of over-drugging. At least 20 percent of the
patients in hospitals are there for iatrogenic diseases
(those diseases caused by the physicians themselves
or the drugs they use). This is a ridiculous record.
This is a condemnation of the United States of America; here we are, a country which can send men to
the moon and bring them back and yet cannot even
find the cure for the common cold.

Classical organized medicine has made wonderful
strides in progress. It has discovered the control of
certain diseases by the use of antibiotics. It has discovered methods of sanitation which have prolonged
the lives of many people. It has discovered methods
of immunization whereby the scourges of poliomyelitis, smallpox, measles and diphtheria are controlled. It has discovered methods of transplanting
hearts or even heart-lung systems from a dead person to one who is about to die. Nothing but praise is
due for such feats of skill and knowledge, if they
succeed.

However, there is a smear on this wonderful record: the search for a cure for cancer. Statistics today are worse for Mr. Average Citizen than ever before. According to the available statistics, one of four now living will develop cancer. It costs Mr. Average Citizen about $15,000 to die of cancer today via the organized medical way.

Many millions, even billions of dollars have been spent in medical research for the cure for cancer. Out of this gigantic complex of cancer research not one really significant discovery has shown its head in the last twenty years. There is much publicity during the fund-raising seasons about how the discovery of the cure of cancer is just around the corner. But which corner?

Actually, there is not a single official study on record of any of the so-called "non-toxic" cancer remedies. A simple double-blind study conducted in an impartial way at one of the great ivory towers of medical knowledge would prove beyond a doubt the validity or not of these remedies. This has not been done. Yet millions of dollars have been spent propagandizing and degrading these remedies as worthless, quackery and dishonest. All the propaganda costs money. The only real explanation seems to be the fear of the public knowing the truth.

The commonly accepted etiological factors in the cause of disease are: age, sex, occupation, residence, past history, family history, heredity, stress and the nutritional pattern. What can a practitioner do about these factors of etiology? Age, sex, past history, family history and heredity are factors that cannot be changed. The occupation and residence of the patient may be manipulated to a certain extent but the results are minimal. Stress or adaption to it can be significantly understood. That leaves only one major factor

xiv

which can be manipulated: the nutritional picture, both present and future. Is it not logical, then, that this potential factor in health should be the prime target area of investigation for the cause and treatment of disease?

Many physicians are beginning to awaken to the fact that what they are doing may be less than the best. They are becoming discouraged. Yet they do not know where to turn. They are frustrated. They wish to do something but are in fear of reprisals. They can afford neither the financial risks nor the reprisals of organizations trying to control them. Rightly so. Yet there is a solution: to learn about nutrition and its relation to health, and then practice it!

Where can one learn about nutrition? There is no place in the ivory towers of organized medicine. There is a dearth of teaching in the contemporary medical schools. There is no real authority to follow.

This book, A New Breed of Doctor, is an attempt to be a beacon light for those who wish to walk in the paths of nutritional know-how. The information presented is specific enough to provide basic working hypotheses for physicians. It is also practical enough for use in the home by the layman. I hope it will be a turning point for both.

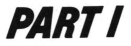

CHAPTER I

THINKING NUTRITIONALLY

Definition

"THINKING NUTRITIONALLY" is an unusual term, and yet the concept behind it is used every day. What it means and what it does not mean are important factors to be considered. It is a positive, body-building program based upon providing an adequacy of the proper nutrients and the elimination of adverse elements whereby overall harmony develops within the body.

What nutritional thinking does not mean is important. Nutrition is not to be confused with ordinary diet. Nutrition does not mean "meat, potatoes, carrots, vegetables and plenty of them." Nor does abundance of food mean that it is adequate for body building. "A good nutritious diet" is a standard statement of nomenclature used in medical schools. As we doctors are taught about diseases and their treatments, the discourse on therapy usually starts with these words: "Recommend a good, nutritious diet." The sad part is, these words are never defined. It is left up to the individual medical student to determine what he thinks the words mean. It is forgotten upon graduation. Another cliché, "I eat all I want, whatever I want, and whenever I want," certainly is not thinking nutritionally. The body of modern man does *not* know instinctively what it needs nutritionally. The usual reaction is to reach for the handiest or habit-forming food. The chances are, in modern society, the handy food is a nonnutritious food and will not solve the need even though it does fill the stomach. Habit-forming foods include salt, coffee, sugar, alcohol and other man-made foods. The more one indulges, the more one wants. Thus, habit, not "wisdom of the body," creates a continuous demand for them, usually to the detriment of health.

The Whole Man

The whole man is composed of numerous distinct units. The smallest integral part of the body is the cell. The cells are grouped together into glands and organs. The glands and organs are arranged into systems. Finally, the whole group of systems is organized to comprise the whole body. The function of the whole body is reflected in the function of the separate parts. For instance, the heartogram and the phonocardiogram do reflect the function of the body as a whole even though they only record actions of the heart. Likewise, a backache reacts on the stamina of the individual: thus, there is a very definite, positive correlation between complaints and diseases. In other words, the whole body is reflected even in simple complaints, regardless of what or where these complaints are.

Whole Needs

Whole bodies have whole needs. There are some seventy or more known nutrients needed by the body for proper function. Different organs and structures have different nutritional appetites. For energy production the brain has an almost exclusive appetite for carbohydrates. Other parts of the body have greater need for protein and fats as well as the carbohydrates. Only whole natural foods can provide *all* the basic nutrients. Whole natural foods are those which are organically grown to a mature state. A processed food is a partial food. For instance, heat destroys vitamin C and lysine, an amino acid (a protein factor). Freezing destroys the precursors of vitamin K. Thus, any type of processing results in unwhole or partial foods; something has been taken away. They cannot nourish the body as they should. If one were to eat only cooked food or frozen food, he would develop deficiency problems because certain nutrients would not be supplied as needed.

There are also basic differences between foods of the same type. Let us take the citrus family, for example. We have oranges, lemons, limes, grapefruits, tangerines and kumquats. All are related, but different. They all contain the vitamin C complex. The vitamin C complex consists of ascorbic acid, chalcone, quercitin, rutin, and pigments such as citrinoids, and hysperidine, carotenoids and bioflavonoids. All of these elements, and maybe more, grouped together comprise the vitamin C complex. They all exist in each of the fruits mentioned but in different percentage ratios. Not only that, but each vitamin C complex is surrounded by "clothes." These are called the naturally associated synergistic factors. Now, in each of these fruits mentioned, there are different concentrations of the vitamin C complex factors and they have different kinds of "clothes." My point is this: if we have need for more vitamin C complex in our bodies, it is more effective to take some of each one of these fruits than it is to take a large amount of any one. Our total body is able to glean a better vitamin C complex ratio of factors from a variety of whole foods than it is from one single whole food.

In relation to whole food, there is another interesting factor: whole foods affect many different structures in the body. Also, many whole foods affect one structure, but one structure is not completely nourished by one food. It needs a diversification or variety of whole or complete foods to affect the whole responses of the body, which consists of many functioning units. When nourished by whole foods, the body has a better chance of achieving overall harmony.

Normalization of Function

Normalization of body function is a result of the complete approach to treatment of the entire (whole) body. Whole foods tend to produce whole cells and tissues, which tend to function normally, thus recreating the whole body. This is total body harmony at its best. However, normalization of the patient and his tissues does have several levels of give-and-take before physical equilibrium is reached. Different organs and systems respond in various degrees and at different rates to any therapy. For instance, nerve tissue responds more slowly than liver or heart tissue. Also, all glands and tissues are not equally sick at the same time. Both of these factors influence the rate of improvement toward a normalization of bodily function through nutritional therapy.

Physical equilibrium represents a complete balance between all nutritional body-building factors: vitamins, minerals, enzymes, amino acids, starches, sugars, fatty acids, coenzymes, water and other elements needed in the body metabolism, with resultant harmony in hormones, endocrines and physiological function.

Population Explosion and Food Pollution

There will be more mouths to feed in the very near future. Therefore, more food will be needed. "Experts" say that we can produce what we are producing today only with the "benefit" of pesticides and synthetic fertilizers. Such fertilizers speed growth but do not allow for full maturity of nutrients in foods. Furthermore, pesticides and synthetic fertilizers are toxic to the human body. They gradually accumulate in the body. Using more chemicals will expedite our demise.

The "American Way" is the rapid consumption of nonrenewable resources. The recent history of our country proves this. The exploitation of the natural resources like trees and oil reserves are prime examples. These resources can never be replaced. We are a waste-oriented society. There will be famine because the synthetic methods of farming will eventually reach the end of the rope. This is where agriculture is beginning to find itself today. Most of the rich farmland has been converted into land for farming less demanding crops because the natural minerals in the soil have been squandered. The soil can no longer produce quality crops as of a few years ago. Farms have also been replaced by housing developments.

There are still some who think that satisfactory harvesting from the ocean is a possibility. Food from the plankton is definitely feasible but we find that plankton cannot grow in polluted water. Some of the ocean areas are already polluted. Actually, the pollutants already cast upon the soils of America will not come to a peak in the oceans until ten years from now. If we think we have pollution now, it will be far worse in ten years, even if we stop polluting this very instant.

Causes of Physical Deterioration

Our life span starts at birth. In actuality, we begin to die the moment we are conceived in our mother's womb. Diseases play an important role in the deterioration of our bodies.

Stress and strain are also factors in deterioration. The physical stresses of overwork and abuse take their toll. Our bodies are worn out a little more with each stress. Anxiety, depression, tension, guilt and paranoia are only a few of the mental attitudes which cause deterioration of the body.

Nutritional stresses definitely can result from eating poor-quality or partial foods. The unacceptable foods are the man-manipulated foods which have been so devitalized that they are no longer nutritious. They are usually fortified so the public can be hoodwinked into thinking that they are the best foods. Since they are made for taste and smell, Mrs. Average Citizen does not seriously consider their lack of nutritional value.

Deliberate, nonnutritive chemical contaminants are used for coloring, acidifying, alkalizing, softening, preserving, often to extend the shelf life of a product. Eye appeal is also a primary promotional objective.

Hereditary factors in human health deterioration should not be overlooked. There are different aspects to these hereditary patterns which can be traced back to racial traits, to family traits and, finally, to parental traits. Genes are inherent within each and every one of us. We are influenced by our ancestors.

So physical deterioration can stem from many causes. The question is, What can we do about it? I do not mean patching up the patient by masking the symptoms of illness with questionable drugs. I do not mean removing an offending organ by surgery, since the patient can't grow another. I do not mean using transplants. History now shows in most cases that one body rejects the organ of another.

What is necessary is to rebuild the body with the substances, found on analyses, which make up that body in the first place. The body is built of many elements besides water. It contains protein, minerals, both organic and inorganic, fats and other elements. Presumably, if the mother has not been denied these elements in her diet, a child is born with a full supply of all elements necessary for health. Soon, however, these elements begin to run out and must be supplied to the body to prevent a deficiency. If they are not supplied, first internal borrowing takes place, then a breakdown occurs somewhere. If a body is denied calcium, for example, it will begin to borrow from various parts of the body. Teeth and bones will suffer. Glands, such as the parathyroids, and nerves, all of which depend upon calcium for efficient functioning, will begin to suffer. The blood suffers. We can prevent the loss of calcium and other elements needed for smooth body functioning by providing the body with a constant supply of them in our diets. The body can then choose what it needs, and it does, and can thus prevent illness or help to hea' itself. Regrowth of tissues and rebuilding bones and teeth from raw material are not science fiction. I have seen it work.

How are these elements obtained by the body? Very simple: through whole, natural food or natural supplements concentrated from such food. *This is the concept of nutrition.* The idea is relatively new. The surface of the science of nutrition has barely been scratched. Food is being analyzed by the laboratories to reveal a growing number of the elements found in a healthy body. A few are known; many are as yet unknown. But it makes no difference. Nature knows, and natural foods contain them all, providing nature has not been altered by man. Man loves to tear natural food apart, add disturbing contaminants, subtract important nutrients or synthesize single factors—which are not the same as those produced by nature. Nature grows nutrients not singly but in combination, each cooperating with the others. Foods are complex substances.

These elements or nutrients are known to the public as vitamins, minerals, amino acids, and so on. Truly they are the building blocks of health. Early man was far healthier than modern man. He lived on these substances in the natural state. He nourished his body with them. He may have suffered from cold or heat. He may have been attacked by a savage beast. He may have been wounded by a poisoned Indian arrow. But he did not have the host of chronic illnesses, such as heart disease, cancer, diabetes and other deficiency or poisoning diseases, so much in evidence today and which are caused by contaminants deliberately added to food.

Brainwashing is a common curse in our civilization. It can be political. It can also be commercial. Those of you who have been warned that nutrition is quackery would do well to look behind the scenes. Who is benefiting from this propaganda? The manufacturer? The distributor? The political machinery? The doctor? My answer is yes. The patient? No. Yet, if you will be honest, intelligent and objective, you will admit that the nutritional concept, though perhaps not the entire answer to health, does have merit. It does make sense.

If you are a patient, you may know more about nutrition than your doctor. Nutritional information is beginning to sweep the world like a prairie fire because it does make sense. People are becoming well as a result. They are looking for a doctor who understands the nutritional concept. There are practically none.

If you are a doctor and if you will catch up with the demands of the public, your future will be far more assured than ever before. You will again achieve that image of respect once accorded you in yesteryear. You will truly satisfy the requirements of your Oath of Hippocrates. Best of all, you will get, and keep, most of your patients well. Your services will be in great demand. I know, because it happened to me. If I can do it, you, too, can do it.

The following chapters will show you how.

CHAPTER II

APPROACHES TO TREATMENT

THE TREATMENT of sick people has always been a topic of great interest. Out of this have been born the different disciplines in the practice of medicine. The Allopathic physician is one who uses large doses of drugs, as well as surgery. The most important aspect of his technique rests upon the diagnosis. Without a diagnosis, he can do practically nothing; he is utterly lost. The Homeopathic physician explores the infinitesimal details of the patient's symptoms and history. From these, he prescribes minute dosages of various substances to effect a cure. The Osteopathic physician uses massage, physiotherapy, corrective exercises and manipulations. He also uses supplements. In this day and age, he is also using surgery and drugs because he is being taken over by the Allopathic group. The Chiropractic physician uses manipulation, physiotherapy and diet. The Nutritionist uses diet and supplements: vitamins, minerals, enzymes, herbs and cytotrophins. The Naturopathic physician uses natural methods including diet, vitamins, minerals, enzymes, herbs, colonics and exercises. Finally, there is the Eclectic physician. He takes from all disciplines what he thinks to be the best and combines them into a system of his own. This is the true individualist. He thinks for himself. Which is the best method? The patient's response must be the answer.

Modes of Patient Management

There are three different modes of approach to patient management: preventive, corrective and therapeutic. Nutrition is an essential factor in each of these methods; however, it is not the only factor. Let us analyze these different categories.

Preventive Measures

Preventive measures are designed to maintain health before deterioration takes place. This method includes exercise, correct nutrition and thought. Exercise of all types should be acceptable to the patient's needs. It should also be pleasurable to him. Walking, swimming, bowling, tennis, jumping rope, golf (minus riding in a cart), gardening, or gymnastics are good possibilities. Housework for women is out. This, and any other exercises not enjoyed, may create more tension than relaxation and thus defeat its purpose. Exercise by itself does not cure disease but it certainly helps in rebuilding damaged tissues when adequate nutrition is present. The reason: it stirs up circulation and helps distribute nutrients to all parts of the body.

Nutrition and supplements are used for prevention, to maintain the status quo. Good eating habits are developed; adequate chewing, good digestion, and timing and adequacy of the meals are also important.

Thought patterns are fundamental for the future normalcy of bodily function. Emotional stress can actually cause congestion in various parts of the body, or seal them off from adequate blood and nutrient supply and cause a variety of diseases, as proven by Hans Selye, M.D.

Corrective Treatment

Specially designed exercises are employed in corrective treatment and can be added to a regular regimen to remedy problems. Physiotherapy is also used for correction. Specific tissues or structures are stimulated for a particular reason.

Corrective nutrition has a different aim than that of prevention or maintenance of health. The diet may be used to detoxify. This may be through a temporary juice fast or a diet of one or two foods only, preferably all raw. A total water fast is risky because it may release stored poisons (pesticides and others) into the blood stream too rapidly and can cause self-poisoning. It has, in some cases, led to serious illness or death. After the body is detoxified, an overall nutritional regime can be gradually introduced. This is discussed elsewhere in greater detail.

Special attention to the digestive capacity is a must. How much hydrochloric acid, pepsin, bile and pancreatic enzymes are present? Supplements are also used generously to get the most response out of the body and are selected for specific purposes. Certain deficient or disturbed tissues require specific supplements. Protomorphogens (substances derived from glands) are used to enhance the normal functions of the various glands and tissues. Foods and tissues should be organic and natural. Supplements should be stabilized vacuum-dehydrated food products, often combined with herbs and enzymes. Surgery should be used only as an emergency corrective measure after natural methods have first been tried; one should never be too quick with the knife.

Therapeutic Measures

Therapeutic measures are aimed at abnormal states, which include both acute and chronic cases.

One should be sure that the fundamental nutritional functions of the body are performing properly. These include proper nutrient intake, good digestion, adequate assimilation, good liver function, extensive distribution to all tissues by exercise as well as good heart and blood vessels, perfect metabolism and, finally, optimal elimination. When all these functions are operating properly, good health results without need for further treatment. The goal, therefore, is to get these functions to return to normal. Various methods can be used. Drugs and chemotherapy, even synthetic vitamins, have a role to play. Some drugs as well as synthetic vitamins do force reactions to take place in the body. Neither drug nor synthetic vitamin can be taken without paying a price, however. Continued use of both drugs or synthetic vitamins may be likened to whipping a tired horse. The "price" is right only if the circumstances warrant the risk of administration.

Therapeutic surgery may be a life-saving measure. It is performed for hemorrhage, for example, and trauma where life is endangered.

Nutritional methods are used in a therapeutic manner for detoxification and rebuilding. Here there is even stricter dietary control and no room for laxity. The diet must be *exact* to accomplish the needs of the situation. The building blocks of repair must be supplied by the diet or supplements if the body is expected to do the repairing. Total foods build total bodies.

An optimal amount of supplements is needed. They are to be taken for a long enough period of time and in large enough dosage to accomplish the task. Physiotherapy and exercises are prescribed in a specific manner, too.

Total gland preparations, called desiccated glandular substances, are extremely helpful. They provide protein and fat components extracted specifically from the gland in question. They cause the glands to respond as well as providing more protein for metabolism. The nucleoprotein extracts of cells, called cytotrophic extracts or protomorphogens, are used with the aim of specific glandular stimulation. Protomorphogens provide specific growth determinants and help the function of the glands to return to normal whether over or underactive.

Avoid misuse of therapeutic tools. X-ray and other types of radiation can be overused, causing burns which may become malignant. Surgical intervention before adequate trial of other methods can also be a detriment; for example, the use of heart transplant techniques *before* an adequate trial of basic nutritional methods may be likened to putting the cart before the horse.

Nutritional medicine is a tool to be used in *all* categories of therapy. Not to use nutritional support during times of extraordinary stress can be likened to a professional football player wearing a bathing suit rather than a football uniform to do his thing.

Nutritional Tools

Nutritional tools must be chosen with great discrimination. First, avoid adulterated foods. "Pure" foods, according to the law, do not have to be pure natural foods. For instance, legally, pure peanut butter needs only to be 92 percent naturally pure. The other 8 percent can be dyes, flavors, fillers, sugar, etc. "Pure" peanut butter does not have to be made from whole nuts. It can be made from broken or culled pieces of nuts. These fragmented pieces are probably rancid even before the peanut butter is made. Adulterated foods also contain preservatives, such as sodium propionate. As soon as some nonfood element like sodium propionate is added for preservative purposes the food is no longer pure from a nutritional point of view. Certain foods, such as soft drinks, low-calorie soft drinks and different kinds of special foods, even those often recommended for diabetics, are deliberately chemicalized. Even though they lower calories or eliminate sugar from the diet, they do not nourish the body as natural foods do.

Deceptive Labeling

Be careful about deceptive labeling! For instance, one label says "organic carrot juice and other juices." Now, this sounds reasonable until you analyze it. Actually, only the carrot juice is organic; not the other juices. A juice *drink,* containing water, sugar and chemicals, is not juice at all! It is a hodgepodge of nonnutritive substances designed only to sell, not to nourish. Unless you read labels carefully, you can be confused, and the expected health results will not be forthcoming.

Devitalized Foods

Avoid devitalized foods. Such foods are processed, the nutrients are removed and then put on the market as food. Such things as flakes of corn, white sugar, white flour, white rice and hydrogenated oils are all devitalized. The living nutrients have been removed in order to retard spoilage and extend shelf life for the seller. A few synthetic nutrients may sometimes be added to the product so that advertising can say that this food can help your body grow twelve different ways, or some such advertising gimmick. Actually this is brainwashing. Seventy or more nutrients that should be present may have been removed, and replaced with twelve synthetic nutrients. *No*

man-made substitute is as good as the natural food!
Beware of completely synthetic foods. Man makes
"foods" out of nonfood substances. This is being done
in margarine and shortenings where nonfood oil from
cotton can be converted into a "food." We also hear,
now, about food being constructed from coal tar products to be used in our future astronaut programs. I
shudder at the contemplated future results.

Contaminated Foods

In agriculture there are many chemicals added to
the soil to "protect" the crops from insect pests.
These are long-acting, nonbiodegradable poisons
which persist in the soil and become a part of the
produce. Frankly, they are killing us. Pesticide re-
straining laws have been held up or ignored by manufacturers who scream that pesticides are necessary.
(They now admit their businesses cannot survive if
the poisons are phased out.)

Another publicity story goes like this: "Aldrin, a
deadly pesticide, is banned from use on bananas."
Sounds good. The catch is, Aldrin is rarely, if ever,
used on bananas. Unless you know the facts, you cannot see through the fog of deception. Contamination
also occurs in processing and packaging of foods.
Preservatives are added at the time of freezing to
retard spoilage. Heat is the biggest sterilizer in the
canning process. Some nutrients are heat labile.
Heated foods are not whole foods. The lining of tin
cans can and does cause disease. Even frozen foods
suffer from nutrient loss. Whole, organic, raw produce is preferable and should make up at least 50
percent of the diet.

Hormones in Foods

The use of hormones in livestock today is another

serious health problem. Diethylstilbesterol has been injected into the beef cattle to cause a more rapid weight gain in a shorter period of time. Diethylstilbesterol is also commonly used on human beings, women, today. It is in some brands of "The Pill." If women were to understand what this substance does to animals, they would wisely not want to take it themselves. Even men who work in female-hormone-producing factories develop abnormal breasts and become impotent. So the big deception is on. I speculate that this is one of the reasons why we cannot tell the difference between the silhouettes of young boys and girls in their early teens. Which is more important: human health or more dollars for the farmer?

Sweeteners in Foods

Chemical additives are deliberately added to foods for many reasons. You already know that the cyclamates, saccharine, and other types of chemical sweeteners are contaminants. Public motivation is, of course, commercially encouraged for low calorie food for diabetics and weight watchers. No matter what the reason is, they are still unnecessary contaminants. Chemicals are even added for the aroma they produce. The aroma of freshness of bread can be, and sometimes is, built into the paper wrapping of the bread to make you think the bread is delicious and nutritious. Sometimes the aroma is wafted by atomizing it from behind the supermarket bread counter into the air to attract more unwary buyers!

What sort of controls exist today guaranteeing the organic nature of foods? Legally, there are none. Voluntarily, there are some efforts. *Sun Circle* brand is the result of one effort to locate and to band together trustworthy organic and natural farmers and their produce under one brand label. This is based upon the individual integrity of the persons sponsoring the program. I can vouch for them. The foods are trustworthy. *Sunshine Valley* products are another attempt to produce quality nutritional foods. These foods, often in supplement form, have been processed by vacuum dehydration and preserved by natural methods and the use of herbs so that they do not lose their nutritional value. Chico San foods are also excellent and, again, the quality is guaranteed on the basis of the integrity of the manufacturer. Do not believe all labels just because you see them in health food stores. There are many good products found in health food stores that are not available elsewhere. There are also a few questionable items.

A Positive Approach to Nutrition

The major positive nutritional concept is to eat foods which spoil, but eat them before they do. Vine or tree-ripened produce is best. These products are supersaturated with the nutrients that develop in them during the last few hours while they remain on the vine or tree. It is wise to eat a variety of whole foods, including most seeds, for the best effects on the whole body. Seeds contain the life of the plant. You should eat the seeds of apples, watermelon and citrus fruits. Seeds are nutritionally important. The only part of an organic apple to be thrown away is the stem.

The foods should be organic and natural. Nutritionally, this means that the produce has been grown by organic methods, including using natural fertilizers and without chemical sprays. "Natural" means that the food is "from a living source" rather than a synthetic source. Here again, be alert to labeling, because "from a living source" could include the coal tar products, since coal tar reserves were once living organisms. The organic and natural concept means a whole natural, unadulterated living food.

Today, when there is a sudden explosion of available health foods, one must be very cautious. Due to sudden demand, "organic food" is being prostituted. Stick to the people who have established voluntary controls and a reputation of trustworthiness. As mentioned before, *Sun Circle* brands, *Sunshine Valley* and *Chico San* products are trustworthy insofar as the natural and organic qualities of the products are concerned. Fortunately, there is a big effort now to establish criteria and to organize the organic farmers who qualify into some sort of federation. Information on this project can be obtained from *Prevention* magazine, Emmaus, Pennsylvania.

How Other Contaminants Invade the Body

The Lungs

Many contaminants, like smog, are airborne and invade the lungs. There are always minute leaks in gas appliances. These leaks are enough to cause illness in some susceptible people.

Other contaminants that enter the body through the lungs come from the pressure containers used for hair sprays, deodorants, furniture polish, insecticides, etc.

Agricultural sprays get into the atmosphere and are inhaled by people. The most dangerous method of application is by airplane. There is much uncontrollable drift.

Nicotine is a contaminant entering our body through the lungs. We do not have to be a smoker to be inflicted with the effects of nicotine. The presence of one smoker in a room contaminates the atmosphere. One cigarette, it is calculated, wastes approximately 25 milligrams of vitamin C from the smoker's body resources. When the official minimum daily requirement is considered to be 60 milligrams of vitamin C per day, one can easily see what a very few cigarettes will do.

Before you pick up that next cigarette, read this: the July 1971 issue of *Reader's Digest* has an excellent article packed with facts and figures on the effects of smoking on health. It states that cigarettes cause miscarriages and stillbirths, defects in children, chronic bronchitis, pulmonary emphysema, heart trouble, lung cancer, peptic ulcers, blindness and gingivitis. When confronted with such information, a typical smoker laughs nervously and utters an immature reply, such as, "At least I'll die happy." But smokers aren't happy when they gasp for oxygen every day for years. They don't think it's funny when children are either born with serious defects or are stillborn. And after a few short years their widows and orphaned children are *not* laughing. Still dying for a smoke? Read the article, friends.

Insect repellent is put into paints, carpets and wallpaper. Continued breathing in a room so treated can be hazardous. Insect strips are also dangerous.

These are some of the examples of the chemicalization of our environment today. There are industrial solvents and chemicals of all types to which mankind is exposed continuously. My examples have barely scratched the surface.

The Gastrointestinal Tract

The gastrointestinal tract remains a major source of ingress of chemicals into the system. The most common source is adulterated foods which contain suspect additives: softeners, colorings, flavorings, extenders, preservatives, drugs, alkalizers, acidifiers, hormones, pesticides and many others, all added for commercial gain but sold to the public under the guise of "protecting our food." There are over 2,500 different chemicals allowed in our food and about 8,000 contaminants in our total environment which we can breathe, drink, eat or touch. Some are potent poisons, others are less active. All are abnormal to the human body and must be excreted or neutralized. Disease, even death, can result from our chemicalization. The man-made pseudofoods are eaten everywhere.

Other contaminants in food are chlorinated and, indirectly, soft water. Chlorine is a poison in this form which kills enzymes as well as germs. Water softeners remove hard minerals, thus causing an excessive intake of sodium which predisposes to more heart trouble. Distilled water contains no minerals, which are already in short supply. We deliberately put drugs and chemicals into our mouths. The toothpastes we use are loaded with chemicals. Just listen to the advertisements on TV. The fluorides for stronger teeth and germ-killing mouth washes are chemicals. Chemicals are poisons in certain dosages. These are partly swallowed as well as being absorbed directly through the mucous membrane of the mouth. Either way, they are chemical contaminants to our bodies, thus adding to the overall stress problem. Drip, drip, drip and pretty soon we have a bucketful.

The Skin

Contaminants can get into the body through the skin. The skin is a living organ and absorbs substances through local applications. The skin is normally acid. Soaps are usually alkaline; therefore, a potential problem. The more soap used, the more problems will result. Some soaps, shampoos, enzymes, hand creams, lotions and shaves are so harsh that we would never knowingly put them on our hands. Yet we may use them as a shampoo, for instance, or a facial cleanser, because of commercial motivation. There are hair products identified as "squeaky clean," the "fluffy waviness" or the "stay-put" product. These are propaganda phrases that have nothing to do with the basic health and nutrition of the hair. Perfumes are chemical substances and are very concentrated. The natural perfumes are preferred to the synthetics but they are all concentrated chemicals. Many people are allergic to these chemicals.

Our clothes represent a source of skin contamination. The concept of "stay-pressed" for trousers is accomplished by the use of chemicals. Moth-proofing to save the clothes from the ravages of moths is accomplished by the use of chemicals. Self-help dry-cleaning of clothes is a very complicated chemical process these days. Fumes inhaled while taking the clothes home in a closed car have caused death. There are also many methods of skin contamination through our clothes. In the household, moth-proofing is put into the cloth that is used for upholstering furniture and in carpeting.

The Liver

The liver acts as a filter for the body. It absorbs and stores poisons. The liver detoxifies the blood by screening out debris and waste products.

Another function of the liver is to make nutrients available for tissue use. Some substances, as they are taken into the body, are not useable by the tissues and must be first chemically converted into available nutrients by the liver. The liver also acts as a storage house for some nutrients so that they can be released as needed.

The liver does a gigantic job and needs all the help it can get. It needs no added burdens. One method of helping a sluggish liver is to use a temporary detoxifying diet. Another is to give the patient liver cytotrophic extract or protomorphogen therapy. Whole liver extracts may be in the form of desiccated liver which has not been exposed to pesticides or other contaminants and processed at low heat so as not to destroy valuable nutrients. The liver is stimulated by its own cytotrophic extract. Liver cytotrophins taken orally go to the local cells of the liver and stimulate them to become more normal in their function. There are also certain herbs which stimulate liver function. These should be used routinely. I personally believe that patients do not become ill unless they have a weakness of the liver even though it cannot be proven in the laboratory. Many times we use a yardstick to measure millimeters; laboratory tests are frequently too gross when it comes to the finer points of diagnosis.

Atomic Radiation

Radiation in our atmosphere today is an extremely vital problem. Not only do we have natural radiation from the cosmos but we have man-made radiation. We know very definitely about X rays and radioactive materials used in medical circles. These are dangerous and respected as such. The atomic reactors as contemplated for the production of electrical energy throughout our country today are without a reasonable doubt sources of danger. The very nature of the atomic reaction means that there is production of radioactive material. This radioactive material can be disposed of in different manners. It can be blown into the air, dumped into waste waters or held in solid form and disposed of later in another way. No matter how energy is produced by the atomic reactors, atomic wastes are by-products. *These atomic waste by-products are a danger to mankind.* We must understand the problems involved and solve them before we become overwhelmed by the radioactive atomic wastes. There are no known "safety factors" concerning atomic radiation which are known to be safe. Microwave towers and ovens also emit radiation of significant degree.

Some Suggested Solutions

1. Encourage educational campaigns, on all levels of school and through newspapers, periodicals, television and radio, to be designed to tell the truth to all. Nutritional truths should be an integral part of the way of life. Such programs should become a popular topic of discussion and as commonplace as the sport page or fashions.

2. Redirect the goal of the Federal Food and Drug Administration (FDA). The original intent of the organization must be reinstated to protect the people, to encourage really pure foods, vitamins, and food supplements and to curb worthless and noxious drugs. Somehow, bureaucracy has gotten out of control and these goals have been lost.

3. Pass anti-pollution laws with teeth in them and with loopholes taken out so that individuals and corporations cannot abuse the privilege of living in the twentieth century. Voluntary or intraindustry controls are apparently useless.

4. Recycle nitrogenous wastes as a practical, realistic solution for disposing of a problem and creating a blessing at the same time. Not only will it result in the production of compost, but it will

also help purify the water.

5. Use vacuum dehydration in food preservation and supplement production. This is very valuable and should be used much more extensively. Food produced in this manner emphasizes the maximum of ripeness and maturation when converted into a stabilized product that retains nutrients. The food is virtually maintained and preserved with enzymes and herbs which are perfectly normal as foods.

6. Utilize seed sprouts in our diet. Sprouts are the early small growth from seeds. The nutritional value of one tiny radish sprout with two little leaves, for instance, is more complete than the mature radish. Sprouts represent the vigor of life.

7. Use herbs. Herbs are available in local areas. It is necessary to study herb books to learn which ones, how and when to use them. Many are very effective. They have been used for centuries. They are easily available and are inexpensive. However, the FDA persecutes anyone who states the value of an herb on its label or makes any claims for it. Some are even being banned.

8. Explore the hazards of the use of birth control measures. It is a desperate situation. The use of the intrauterine device, or IUD, is less than satisfactory. The very mechanism, notably keeping the uterus in a state of chronic inflammation so that the egg will not become implanted, is not healthful. Chronic infections which may result are never healthful. The use of "The Pill," which manipulates the female endocrine function, is functionally satisfactory and yet it is not 100 percent perfect. There are too many complications. I am thoroughly against the use of "The Pill." Anything that can cause that kind of hormonal disturbance in the system can and does cause other kinds of hormonal imbalances and tissue

reactions. There are serious side effects to be considered. The use of contraceptives appears to be something pretty much in the past and judged inconvenient. Foams can be used and are very satisfactory with the one exception that they, too, are chemical and are absorbed into the system from the vaginal tract.

These are some suggested solutions to many of the problems that we face. No doubt there will be more problems. Public apathy towards these problems is no longer acceptable. It is your problem and mine. We are obligated to take action.

How and why I—the son of an orthodox physician —changed from what I was originally, a physician, trained in orthodox procedures, to what I am today? I will tell you about it in the following chapters. I hope my story will help other doctors, and I hope it will also help patients.

CHAPTER III

MY PERSONAL INITIATION

Art's Story

"HOW AM I doing, Doc?" Art asked as I examined him. This seemed to be an unnecessary question because his pulse was fine, his blood pressure good, he had no pain and he was back on the job. All of this after having suffered a coronary heart attack a few months before. I told him these things as I reassured him.

He looked at me and said, "I've done all you ordered, but I've done something else too." This led to a discussion about a food supplement which he had been taking in addition to what I had given him and culminated in a purchase amounting to $24.96, not for Art, but for me!

His coronary attack had been relatively mild; yet no illness is mild when it concerns the heart. I had followed the usual medical management in his case, with one exception: I had not given him anticoagulants. This was a form of treatment about which I had never been really convinced. Among other things used in the management of his case were vitamin B-12 injections and a high potency synthetic vitamin product from the drugstore. He had added natural and organic vitamins to the program on his own and felt that this had helped his recovery.

To make a long story short, I tossed the box of supplements I bought, recommended by Art, onto a shelf in the office and didn't pay further attention to it.

27

But it was there. I had paid out $24.96. It finally dawned on me that this was a loss of money unless I put it to use. So the girls at the office and I started to take the tablets, one yellow and two green, three times daily. We began to feel better; we had a little more energy; we could get our work done easier. My wife became suspicious when she noticed that I was singing in the shower in the mornings. She wanted to know why. I brought some vitamins home and gave them to her and our daughters. The entire family soon felt better. We became convinced of the value of the natural nutritional supplements, as compared to the synthetic types.

A question prodded me: how could such a vitamin mineral tablet do anything for me? I was already taking a 5x potency synthetic vitamin-mineral product, yet I got added benefits by taking this organic-natural product of relatively small potency. I was very skeptical at this point. I wondered why this was so. I began to search in earnest, and eventually learned some surprising things.

Incident at Medical School

In retrospect, I remembered a time when I was on the medical ward while I was a student in medical school. A heart patient was being discussed and the professor in charge was saying that the treatment of this case should actually have started some ten years before. By this he meant that, if the patient had taken care of himself properly during the preceding years, he would probably have avoided this particular heart attack. This now became a nagging thought while I was pondering Art's problem.

Swanie's Story

At this time we had a pair of dachshund dogs. Mamie and Ike were their names, so you know the vintage. These dogs were very dear to us and the children liked them very much. Suddenly, one evening, Mamie developed paralysis in her hindquarters. She could not jump onto the chair as usual. We checked with the veterinarian. He was helpless. We tried to take care of her at home but it soon became impossible. We had to have Mamie put to sleep. This was a big tragedy to the family because we all loved her.

It was not long before another female dachshund joined our family. This dog, Swanie, was two and a half years old. She was in good health, we fed her a good nutritious diet consisting of the best canned foods available for dogs, but, surprisingly, six months later there was a recurrence of the same dramatic scene. She, too, developed paralysis in the hindquarters. We rushed her to the veterinarian, who suggested rest and sedation. We watched as her condition deteriorated.

Fortunately a dentist friend happened along who said, "Take her home and I'll tell you what to do." This friend outlined a basic nutritional program. We gave her many different kinds of vitamins, including B-12 shots. We put hot packs on her hindquarters. The hot packs caused a profuse sweating. Now I know dogs are not supposed to sweat, but this dog was dripping wet and the odor was extremely offensive; we could scarcely go into the room. However, she gradually improved. As the improvement gained momentum the odorous condition decreased. Ultimately, she made about a 90 percent recovery. She lived for another five years after this episode and was able to run up and down hills and chase the other dogs without serious difficulty. There was only about a 10 percent residual paralysis in her muscles. Later her leg was broken when she was accidentally thrown off an orchard truck. In spite of this leg with the cast on it, she was running around and taking care of her business. Several years later she died slowly of heart and kidney failure following the use of flea collars. More about this later.

Challenging Thoughts

These experiences produced challenging thoughts which had to be integrated into my life. How could incurable conditions be almost cured by nutritional methods? I had to know. How could I practice medicine, aware that something like this was happening and available without understanding the basic principles? I became convinced that my patients were suffering because of my lack of knowledge.

How Naïvete Caused My Downfall

While pondering along these lines, my major concern was to be able to deliver better services to my patients. I was not a knight in shining armor. I was no crusader. Such ideas never occurred to me. I had always believed that good, better and best results in patient management were the goals of medical practice. To my chagrin, as you will see, I soon discovered that politics were much more important.

I had embarked on a self-teaching program. True, I made errors while learning. There was no formal education available; I could not go back to school to learn nutritional medicine because there was no such course. I had to learn on my own by reading and talking to people. One medical physician in southern California was very valuable to me. He also had been trained in an orthodox medical school and, as I had, had practiced accordingly for a number of years. But he, too, experienced a challenge.

His wife was a nutritional laboratory researcher. When he witnessed the surprising results she produced in test animals, using nutritional substances rather than drugs, he decided to test some of these same nutritional substances on his patients. The results were very dramatic. He began using more and more nutritional therapy. He, too, began to read, research and learn more about nutrition until today he is a walking encyclopedia on the subject. He had also been forced to teach himself, since there was no other source of knowledge. By the time I met him, he had been practicing nutritional therapy for a number of years and had developed a fantastic approach to the problem. He shared his knowledge with me. He answered my questions. He showed me what and how he practiced. He helped me to interpret findings and results. It was very gratifying and enormously helpful to meet such a man.

Disgruntled Colleagues

During this learning phase some of my patients misinterpreted results. Sometimes while they were detoxifying on my program they suffered disturbing effects. They concluded these results were due to the vitamins I recommended rather than to the beneficial effect of the body being cleansed. My colleagues deliberately misinterpreted what I was doing and did not want to learn anything about nutritional methods. At one medical society meeting, I had the audacity to mention to an eye specialist that I thought that I was getting some good response in the treatment of a case of cataracts by nutritional methods. Without asking for facts, he said simply, "If you're not careful, I'll have to report you to the society." My colleagues evidently had only one thought in mind, which was how to stop such heresy!

Medical Society Action

Then came the blow. I was called on the carpet by

medical authorities. When I tried to present my views, there was no give-and-take discussion allowed. Yet there was plenty of discussion when I was absent as they talked about me and my efforts. Some formal hearings finally were held as the situation began to come to a head. In one particular local medical grievance committee meeting, I presented my side of the story. It is recorded on my tape. After my presentation they asked me to leave the meeting. Their discussion then took place. I was later told that the findings were against me. I appealed the findings to the state medical level. At the state-level meeting I noticed some papers were being passed out to the committee members. I asked, "What's that?" They answered that it was a report of what happened at the previous hearing.

I said, "Well, if this is evidence against me, I should have a chance to see it." With much persuasion, I was finally able to see this document. It was supposed to be a verbatim transcript of the former meeting, which I had also recorded on my tape. This transcript was so distorted that not one line of it, and it consisted of some twenty-two pages, was accurate according to what had actually happened. I have both documents in my possession at the present time.

Needless to say, the result of that committee hearing, too, was against me. They were not the least bit interested in straightening out the differences between the printed document and what had really transpired. They were forced to have a hearing and that's what they had. What really took place was not important, especially the truth of the situation. By their constitution they were forced to allow a hearing. This they did and that was all. The result of the hearing was a decision against me. They apparently had been ordered by higher-ups to crucify me. They tried. They are still trying.

The climax of the whole situation was my expulsion from the medical society "because of unethical conduct." This occurred in March 1962 and was a shock to me and to my family. It was announced to my community on Sunday morning on the first page of the local newspaper.

Actually, this excommunication was for no other offense or "crime" than doing something "different" from the rules made and enforced by the medical organization dictatorship. What I had learned and the nutritional substances I was using with my patients were getting better, more lasting and safer results than the drugs I had previously used. I felt I was making a far greater contribution to the permanent health of my patients. They began to think so, too. As one patient told another, my practice started to grow. Instead of my punishment for "heresy" being the end of my practice, as my detractors had planned, it became a turning point. I stuck it out, refused to be turned out of my profession and became more determined than ever, medical society membership notwithstanding, to help my patients achieve better health through nutritional medicine.

Friends Become Aware

My enemies put every stumbling block they could think of in my way. They continue to do so. My friends, who at first had not been aware of me, because of the deliberately planned, untrue, and unsavory publicity, discovered me and began to see that I was doing something new, important and helpful. From that point on, my practice began to grow and it has grown ever since. I still realize that I have not found all of the answers, but, after experience with thousands of patients, I have learned a lot and continue to learn more about a new-found and growing science: nutritional therapy.

Side Effects

There were some side effects from no longer being in the local medical society. The California Medical Association and the American Medical Association dropped me on the excuse of nonpayment of dues. I tried to pay directly but these payments were refused because they had to be paid through the local medical society. Since the local medical society would not accept my dues, the AMA and the CMA dropped me from membership. Hospital privileges were denied me because the bylaws of the staffs of the various local hospitals require that staff physicians be a member of the local medical society. This was a sad loss because there always comes a time in a physician's experience when he needs to send a patient to the hospital. As I had been in practice for a number of years, there were older patients who were approaching the end of their lives. They would need me, the physician of their choice, when they were passing on, yet I was not allowed to be with them.

Family Reaction

My expulsion from the medical society was also a sad episode in my own medical family. My father had been a successful medical practitioner in our local community. My brother is a specialist in internal medicine and my sister, a trained medical technician, is married to a doctor who is a specialist in otolaryngology. Now, when we get together for family gatherings, we no longer talk about medicine. I am the black sheep of the family. This is truly sad. Even so, my experience proved not to be the end, but the beginning of a new career: a new breed of doctor.

CHAPTER IV

PROGRESS—FULL SPEED AHEAD

My "Guinea Pigs"

As TIME went on new ideas and concepts came to me. Their validity was determined by trial and error. If they seemed to fit in a logical sequence, I tried them on myself, on my family and on the employees in the office. Generally speaking, all were good sports right down the line. There was so much learning to be done. At one time, when I believed my discoveries were original, I started to write a book. Then I discovered others had written books. These books were written by authorities who had many years more experience than I. After all, I was just a neophyte and, by comparison, really had nothing new to say. So much information was already known, researched and documented far beyond my own research. Nevertheless, my investigation has continued throughout the years. If I see some evidence which is contrary to my nutritional training or thinking, I am open-minded to a new concept, no matter how surprising, and test it for validity.

Prince's Story

Prince is another of our dogs. He is a combination of Malemute and German shepherd; a beautiful dog with a wonderful personality. Once he was in a fight with a pack of dogs. He came out second best but put up a good fight. His back and neck were injured.

Although I have had some chiropractic friends work on him with good temporary results, he continues to have some problems.

When we moved to a ranch in 1967, we discovered that Prince had a lot of fleas which he shared with the other dogs. We began using flea collars. We thought the flea problem was under control until, suddenly, Swanie developed toxic reactions to the collars. She eventually died. (Note: For safe flea control, put eucalyptus leaves in dog and cat beds.)

Prince was a little luckier. He merely developed a rash around his neck. Being a younger and healthier dog, his rash simmered for two or three months until suddenly the rash spread over his whole body. The exact cause of the spread was mysterious but the result was an eczematous, weeping, scaly lesion over his whole body. He was losing his hair rapidly. He was a very sick dog. My impression was that he had been poisoned by the flea collars. We started to treat him nutritionally. We gave him various vitamins, minerals, food supplements and cytotrophic extracts just as I now treat my patients. He was taking a handful of pills several times a day. In about three or four days we began to see some improvement. He was aware that we were trying to help him so would usually take the tablets without much fuss. He recovered but his heart showed the strain. He could no longer run up and down the hills or play with the other dogs. He would walk along with us but would huff and puff all the way. Many times he would stay home because it was too much effort to move. Again I resorted to more and different nutritional factors: heart cytotrophin and other vitamins and substances to strengthen heart function. He got better. Four or five years later he still has something of a heart problem but it is under control and he does run with the other dogs.

One day about six months after this episode a lump developed under the skin on his left rib cage. It was the size of my fist. It was movable and firm. It was not a lymph node. This worried me because such things just do not happen without reason. My nutritional diagnosis was that his mineral balance was not what it should be. He was given a preparation of beet-root powder which is organically produced in Germany and is reported to contain all the trace minerals. He was given one teaspoonful per day. Lo and behold, the lump subsided in about two weeks. Unfortunately, we ran out of beet powder for a couple of months. The lump returned. When we resumed the beet powder, the lump went away again and has never returned.

At the present time Prince still suffers from a bit of arthritis. On cold mornings he has trouble getting started. He still runs and chases deer so much at night that it aggravates his gait during the day, especially when he does not want to do something that we want him to do. Again, nutrition had proved helpful where other measures failed.

Preventive Medicine

One of the benefits resulting from my new approach was an improved diagnostic ability. This developed because of a more thorough patient-evaluation routine. Practice makes perfect. To be honest, the more thorough patient analysis was a result of my being afraid of what might be said against me if a medical organization spy were sent into my office. My reasoning was that if my records were more complete than those of my accusers and if I ever had to go to court, they would look rather silly trying to say that my checkup was inferior. They might be able to say that I missed some diagnosis or something similar, but they could not say that I neglected to try to understand the patient's problem.

My nutritional therapy program continued. Word of its beneficial results was spreading. More patients were coming in for consultation because of personal testimonies from others. The effects of the preventive treatment began to develop. I kept looking for possible future problems in order to nip them in' the bud before they became real problems.

Frankly, the results in some patients still utterly amaze me; they are absolutely startling. There are many added fringe benefits, too. Experience in nutrition is highly convincing. I have come to know and believe absolutely that degenerative conditions of the body are usually nutritional in origin. They are the result of localized areas of malnutrition. I have also discovered that early therapy gives the best results. This is only natural. The longer a situation exists, the harder it is to treat, because progressive metabolic damage has taken place.

I also feel that bacterial infections develop because of weakened local tissue integrity due to malnutrition. It is the weakened area that attracts the bacterial infection. For example, why doesn't everyone get cholera, typhoid or smallpox during epidemics? If disease depended only upon the exposure to the microorganism, then everyone should get sick. Since everyone does not get sick, we must say that there is a difference in the individual person insofar as resistance is concerned. The only explanation is better health of the local tissue which is being maintained by good, better or best nutrition.

In actuality, disease syndromes are due to failure of glands, organs, or systems. Hypoglycemia, diabetes, coronary heart attacks, allergic diatheses, colitis, ulcers, and so on are disease syndromes, symptomatic patterns, which are secondary to the failure of particular glands, organs, or systems due to underlying malnutrition. There is also the subclinical problem vs. the clinical. There are the definite clinical manifestations of nutritional diseases, such as scurvy, beriberi, which are manifest; but what about the subclinical conditions which are merely slumbering, waiting to erupt? No illness develops overnight. They develop slowly over a period of time; there must be a subclinical state before the obvious disease condition.

These subclinical manifestations are important and represent the various complaints that are experienced by the patient for which the average doctor can find no cause. They may have no organized symptomatic pattern. It might be a series of subtle aches and pains. Whatever it is, there is no explanation for all these symptoms except an unnoticed state of malnutrition. The doctor may tell the patient, "There is nothing wrong with you," or, "It's all in your mind." But the patient is right; there is something brewing behind the scenes. Before eruption into an actual disease, the patient feels symptoms and knows all is not well.

Predicting the Future

I believe that the practice of medicine, as we know it today, is on the verge of a gigantic upheaval. It will be an ecologic and nutritional revolution. In spite of the wonderful strides made in surgery and medicine, the use of strong drugs or chemicals is overextended. The use of drugs in medical practice has become absurd. Twenty percent or more of the inmates in hospitals are there because of the use of medical drugs. Also, surgery has reached a point where even organized medicine no longer has control. There are many knife-happy surgeons. "Almost-routine" tonsillectomies and adenoidectomies are wrong in principle. Even experts agree on this, yet wholesale operations continue. The knife is used to amputate an appendix when, many times, a little nutritional care would solve the problem. A gallbladder removal because of gallstones could often be avoided if the stones could be made to pass by a few simple nutritional measures. Surgery can accomplish many miraculous things which were not even dreamed of a few decades ago, but it can also be used indiscriminately.

In psychiatry, there are some advancements toward better living. There is also much double-talk. Patients are beginning to find out what is going on behind the scenes and frequently do not like what they see. They, like some doctors, are beginning to rebel against organized medicine. The fight will become more intense.

I also envision that many doctors as well as laymen will become interested in nutritional education, training, and therapy. At the present time there is still no formal educational nutritional facility available. Nutritional wisdom must be acquired through self-education. How one does this is discussed in Chapter VIII.

I have visited several doctors who are doing some sort of nutritional work. These doctors opened their offices and their ideas to me. I visited some in California, New York, Florida and Nebraska. These were some of the key doctors who influenced my thinking.

The success of a doctor's practice of metabolic nutrition hinges upon his experience. His experience is determined by his desire, his study, his application of nutritional knowledge to practice. There must be honesty. There must be a great amount of patient understanding or empathy. Not only is ability important; so also is availability.

Finally, there is the opportunity for application of nutritional knowledge. The medical revolution is an ideal testing ground. Many doctors are beginning to know more about metabolism and nutrition in relation to their own practices of medicine and themselves. They are going to continue to grow. There will be leaders and there will be followers. Eventually nutritional therapy will become a realistic tool.

What will be the outcome of the ecological revolution which is going on right now? No one knows. I do know that big business and big government must pay attention. Doctors must also pay attention or they are going to be left behind. The secret of success in making use of an opportunity is preparedness. If we are prepared when the opportunity comes, it will be a stepping stone to greater success.

Many doctors have long been interested in nutrition in connection with their medical practice. Individually they fear to speak out because they know that organized medicine is able and willing to inflict reprisals. Meanwhile, patients, who are getting fed up, are constantly bombarding them with sound nutritional articles from periodicals, newspapers, and magazines. Some doctors are reading these and available books. Some very serious questions from doctors come to me as a result of my column in *Let's Live Magazine*. They want to know. They are searching.

Purpose of this Book

I hope this book will be a breakthrough and provide a pattern for other doctors. Not only will they see what happened to me but, also, the gratifying results of nutritional medicine on patients. There is one problem which must be faced. We cannot have any more sweeping under the rug of the *scientific* nutritional studies that are being done throughout the world. Nutritional research is being done in a qualified manner by qualified individuals at great personal sacrifice and in increasing numbers of universities. It is being reported and published. Organized medicine tends to hide and ridicule these reports. Nutritional research must be performed in more medical schools which are recognized as authoritative by organized medicine. Nothing is to be gained except a loss of confidence in the doctor or medical organization which refuses to acknowledge scientific laboratory nutritional findings concerning human health.

This is a whole new field for a doctor to explore in depth. He can develop a bright new future for an undreamed-of success in practice while he is truly helping mankind. The doctors who have already started in this new field are swamped. I can personally testify to this. Some are actually turning away patients. The public has taken the bit in its teeth; they are ready for a new breed of doctor and will support him. The old breed of doctor will soon find himself spurned.

CHAPTER V

GETTING WELL NUTRITIONALLY

ONE DAY I was called to see a young lady who was suffering from a sore throat and mouth. My examination confirmed her complaints and I prescribed a large dosage of vitamin C. In discussing the situation with her, I told her that her primary condition was actually a form of scurvy, or vitamin C deficiency. The next day she called to tell me that she had consulted another physician who advised her that she did not suffer from scurvy at all, that it was simply a case of pharyngitis. She believed this other doctor even though she was improving on the vitamin C therapy. She was extremely indignant with my diagnosis and, needless to say, never darkened my door again. People do not like to be told, without proper education, that they suffer from malnutrition. They want to have some sort of respectable diagnosis; it seems to be a status symbol.

There are many different intermediate ailments which are of malnutritional origin. Stomach ulcer, arthritis, allergic tendencies, and many others are examples. If there were no local areas affected by malnutrition, these syndromes would never have developed. They can be multiple in nature, too. For instance, one can be allergic and have an ulcer simultaneously.

Many patients urgently need to be shown the true nature of their illnesses. Most have consulted several practitioners to no avail. The usual advice given is that their illness is in their minds; that there is no physical basis for the symptoms which plague them; that they need the help of a psychiatrist. After my complete metabolic analysis followed by an honest presentation of the facts which I discover, I find patients are usually willing to accept the diagnosis of a deficiency disease. When they understand they accept the diagnosis and cooperate with my therapeutic program. It is the physician's job to educate the patient.

There is now no doubt in my patients' minds that my practice is based upon nutritional therapy; that drugs are used only when absolutely necessary and, even then, only after I have told them why I consider drugs necessary. They know I routinely use diets, vitamins, minerals, herbs and other types of nondrug medications. This is why most of my patients come to me. It is a specialty practice which can be called Metabolic Nutrition.

Malnutrition as a Cause of Disease

It is my opinion that malnutrition is a very definite cause of disease. Localized areas of malnutrition set up susceptible foci, or favorable soil, for the development of degenerative or infectious diseases. Each person has a weak link; this plus his past history, age, sex, occupation, stress, place of residence and hereditary factors determine where the individual patient breaks down first. Slight changes may also be intensified by stress. Conversely, stresses become relatively more severe as the integrity of the cells breaks down. It becomes a vicious circle. All disease entities go through a series of degenerative stages, more or less rapidly, before the actual disease state finally appears.

Nutrition vs. Pharmacology

There is a diametrically opposed difference between the nutritional and the pharmacological approaches in the practice of medicine. In the nutritional corner, the main purpose is to strengthen the normal body functions and the patient's resistance so that diseases can lose their hold. The pharmacological approach is to remove the symptoms. In other words, correct nutrition, which contains the identical intrinsic components of the tissues, helps the tissues to rebuild and repair themselves, thus producing health. Drugs merely remove symptoms and mask the cause. To repeat: for example, an aspirin can stop a headache but it does not remove the cause of a headache.

Penicillin and other antibiotics do kill germs, but the germs are only an intermediate, not a primary, cause of illness. Malnutrition must precede the infection in order to prepare the "soil" for bacterial growth. This is true of plants, animals, and people. Thus, antibiotics do kill germs but do not correct malnutrition.

Sometimes drugs are necessary to knock out resistant germs. This is of value when body defenses are at a low ebb and need quick help in order to fight the disease. Thus, drugs can be used as emergency measures to stop rapid and dangerous deterioration before it is too late. Drugs do not *feed* the cells as nutritional substances do. If drugs must be given, they should be given in combination with nutritional supplements. For instance, antibiotics kill valuable intestinal flora as well as dangerous disease germs. European doctors know this. They supply these friendly bacteria simultaneously with and following the administration of antibiotics. Such benign bacteria appear in soured milks, yogurt, acidophilus culture, and other substances. Remember, too, that antibiotics can create dangerous side effects. All drugs have a toxic level. Antibiotics should be given only if absolutely necessary, and only on a temporary basis. If they can kill germs, they can eventually kill a body in too high a dosage or too prolonged use.

Therapeutic Measures

In illness, or pre-illness, the body needs extra help. Determination of the amount of nutritional supplements, such as vitamins and minerals, is as important as the determination of drug dosage, should the latter be necessary.

When a person is ill, his needs are greater for three reasons. He needs nutrient support for normal basic function of cells, organs and glands. He needs additional nutritional help to correct the damage of certain areas of the body, which is now apparent. And he needs extra help because illness is a time of maximum stress and, therefore, demands more than usual nutritional support.

An essential nutrient is a substance normally found in food which is necessary for life and health. Body analyses show that these same substances are present in healthy humans. During illness, it makes sense that larger doses of these supplements or nutrients extracted from food, as opposed to synthetic nutrients which are incomplete in unknown nutrients, are needed for tissue, organ or gland repair. As the body improves, the dosages can be lowered. When it reaches normal, only the amount of these nutrients for the maintenance of health and the prevention of illness is needed. The body gets more miles per gallon out of the nutrients as the cellular metabolism approaches normal.

Nutritional Measures

In health, carefully chosen whole natural foods, in sufficient variety provided by a different menu thirty days out of every month to assure that *all* nutrients are available, may be enough to maintain health. Few people get this type of diet. Stress is rampant in our civilization. This means more need for nutrients. The nutrients, if extracted from whole unadulterated food, as they should be, are the equivalent of many pounds of food. In nature, vitamins, minerals and amino acids (protein factors) appear together and work together in the body. The body needs them all for health. The familiar injection of vitamin B-12 weekly, for example, is merely a drop in the bucket.

Since heating kills many nutrients, as proven in laboratory tests, a diet should contain at least 50 percent raw food to compensate for losses in cooking. For an elderly person with denture problems or a patient unable to assimilate roughage, these raw foods can be converted into liquids by the use of a blender or juicer. Food thus prepared must be used immediately. Even exposure to the air causes a loss in vitamin C; exposure to light causes a loss of some B vitamins, such as riboflavin or vitamin B-2. Don't take my word for it. The scientists have already discovered this and many more facts about what can happen to tampered foods.

If a person is reasonably well and wants to stay well, he can start out with this type of super food supply alone, without added supplements, and try it on for effect. It may or may not be enough for him. His way of life, the amount of stress he faces, his digestion and his assimilation are all factors which determine how many nutrients his body needs.

Cytotrophic Extracts—Protomorphogens

A cytotrophic extract, or protomorphogen, is different from a dehydrated or desiccated extract. A protomorphogen is a component of the cell. It contains the smallest unit of the gene system that guides the cell into its hereditary form as it grows, develops or repairs itself. Without sufficient protomorphogen content the cell degenerates, becomes senile and dies.

The cytotrophin, or protomorphogen, is derived from the cell by extracting its nucleoprotein factors. The nucleus contains chromosomes, genes, RNA, DNA, and other yet-to-be-discovered factors. In simpler terms, the cytotrophic extracts contain the blueprints for cellular determination.

These extracts are derived, by means of a special process, from tissues, glands and organs. Radioactive tracers show that liver extract, for instance, when fed orally to the body, heads directly for the liver. This is respectively true for other glandular and organ extracts too: eye, brain, kidney, pancreas, heart, or whatever. There is a reactivation toward normal cellular activity when these substances are used.

Natural vs. Synthetic

There is a vast difference between synthetic and natural vitamins and minerals, if the latter are truly natural. In natural food, many factors occur together: vitamins, minerals, amino acids and enzymes, which help the body utilize the nutrients. There are many elements which have already been isolated and discovered; there are many more which have not. For example, in the vitamin B category, years ago we thought B-12 was probably the last to be discovered. We are already up to B-22 and still going. So when you eat natural foods or take supplements derived from them, you are getting all the factors, known and unknown. I find that such natural products yield far better results than synthetics.

Most chemists maintain that, molecule by molecule, synthetic vitamins are identical to natural vitamins. The isolated factor of each may be identical, although newer information even challenges this belief. The synthetic vitamin contains one factor only, or perhaps a man-made combination of a few synthetics, which mixtures are merely a combination of the separate factors, not the whole complex found in natural products. These may be called the naturally associated synergistic factors. The whole family of B, or C or E, vitamins is known as a complex. It is true that research shows that separate factors can effect improvement of certain conditions. The whole complex, however—because of the whole spectrum of nutrients it contains—can do even better. It is this type of product I insist upon.

It is true that a sluggish organ, cell or gland may be temporarily stimulated into action by large amounts of a separate synthetic factor, but, if this is continued too long, it becomes similar to whipping a tired horse. The prolonged action of the synthetics imitates the action of drugs. In other words, they only overstimulate and do not feed.

For those scientists who insist that the isolated synthetic factor is the same as the identical isolated natural factor, I have news for them. Some scientists have found that sensitive crystallizations of natural nutrients can be photographed. These photographs, called chromatograms, look like varicolored snowflakes. When they are compared with chromatograms of synthetic factors of the same nutrient, there is a vast difference in the pattern of each. You can't fool a camera.

Basic Principles of Therapy

The primary aim of therapy is the restoration of

the basic function of the body. Nutrition can play a dramatic part. Knowing and establishing the diagnosis is much less important for the patient than correcting malfunction of the organ or part. Patients may want a name for the condition, but, far more important, they need a cure. If vitamin E helps ailing hearts, and it does, it should be given to the heart patient immediately rather than waiting to establish the diagnosis. In the medical vernacular, this means to let the patient get worse until the diagnosis is obvious. Adequate heart function is vital. One should not risk heart failure by not giving vitamin E just to establish the diagnosis for the insurance carriers or the hospital records.

A case in point is one I remember quite distinctly. A recently retired gentleman had just finished moving his furnishings to my community from the Los Angeles area. He had overexerted himself during the previous few days and was suffering with pains in his chest. Since he had a history of coronary artery disease, it was not hard for him to figure out that he was suffering from a recurrence of his trouble. I was called into the case and concurred with the tentative diagnosis. I gave him intensive emergency heart therapy consisting of Cardiotrophin, a heart cytotrophic extract, and vitamin complexes: Cataplex E, E-2, G and C. These tablets were given to him to chew on a five-minute basis until the pain subsided. The dosage was then gradually reduced over the next several days to a maintenance level. He responded dramatically. There was no recurrence of heart pain from the onset. It was a spectacular success in view of his former history.

A few days later the gentleman's son appeared on the scene and told his father he was not sympathetic with the nutritional program I had used. He arranged a consultation with a specialist. Naturally, there was, by this time, nothing unusual for the specialist to find. He declared the patient to be hale and hearty and said he did not need any treatment. In fact, he stated that the whole nutritional program had been nothing but a farce, totally unnecessary and entirely for self-gain. He would have sung a different tune had he witnessed the patient prior to the treatment. If the cure is made and there is no residual evidence of the disease, a nutritionally ignorant colleague can always claim a misdiagnosis. It is an unavoidable trap in the nutritional practice of medicine.

In case of illness, once the emergency problems are overcome, the follow-up therapy program must be instituted to maintain health. Adequacy of intake of nutrients is imperative. The vitamins, minerals, enzymes and tissue supplements of all types need to be taken orally. Since many of them cannot be manufactured within the body, they must come from supplements derived from outside sources. Fortification is also necessary with elements for proper digestion: enzymes, bile salts, hydrochloric acid and pepsin.

Since the digestive processes are started in the mouth, the food and supplements should be masticated and macerated in the mouth. Digestion continues in the stomach, where the hydrochloric acid and pepsin work. The bile salts and pancreatic enzymes work in the duodenum.

Absorption is another important factor. I can almost guarantee the use of *Comfrey-Pepsin* (a product of Standard Process Laboratories) in this regard. Taken in capsule form, the comfrey causes the pepsin to stick to the walls of the intestinal tract so that the mucous crust can be dissolved. Otherwise, the mucous forms an area for easy putrefaction between itself and the mucosa of the intestinal tract. This is eliminated by the Comfrey-Pepsin, allowing better absorption of nutrients and preventing absorption of alimentary putrefactive contaminants.

Liver: The Vital Organ

The liver is the key organ for good health. If this organ is not doing its job, the rest of the body suffers. The function of the liver is multiple. There are some three hundred different functions normally performed by the liver. I assume liver damage is present whether or not it can be proven by laboratory methods.

Merely prescribing or taking nutrients is not enough. In addition to proper digestion, the nutrients must be delivered to the tissues in order to be available for cellular use. This demands a good cardiovascular system. If the heart is not functioning well, the delivery system is inadequate. The health of the arteries, veins, capillaries and lymphatics also influences heart action and delivery of nutrients.

When the nutrients eventually reach the cellular level, metabolic repair is speeded. There must also be an adequacy of oxygen, cytotrophins, vitamins, minerals and enzymes; *all* the nutrients! All the various needed nutrients must be present at the time the reaction takes place. The cell does not know that item X will be eaten at the next meal; the cell wants it now. If it is not present, either the reaction does not take place or it takes place in a distorted manner. In either case, it is less than good and is reflected in cellular malfunction.

Finally, there is the matter of excretion of waste products. This is extremely important since the accumulation of waste products can and will poison the cells and the whole body. Toxins must be eliminated by means of a detoxification process.

Corrections in metabolism are to be made wherever indicated regardless of the primary diagnosis. In the overall approach the patient is treated not just as a heart or a left nostril, but as a total entity, with each part interrelated with the other.

Adverse Reactions

Occasionally there are some undesirable reactions to nutritional therapy. One should not give up and throw the baby away with the bathwater. Correct reanalyses and open-minded assessment is needed at this point. For instance, the synthetic vitamins can and sometimes do cause undesirable reactions. Synthetic vitamin D and ergosterol are examples. A hasty misinterpretation could throw blame on the nutritional therapy by those who do not know that synthetics are not a true part of nutritional therapy. Synthetics are nonnatural elements which are really drugs by vitamin names. As I have said before, they work as drugs, not as nutrients.

There are even some true allergic reactions to natural vitamin complexes. Some people are allergic to strawberries, others to cucumbers. Yet allergies to natural nutritional supplements are more rare than expected. In fact, the very items which might cause reactions are frequently the specific items needed for a cure. This type of reaction is commonly called a histamine reaction. It is a sign of local tissue and cellular starvation which happens when previous injury is already present. Most, if not all, allergic manifestations are eventually eliminated as the cells are restored to their normal nutritional metabolism. However, the tissues may be so deteriorated that they cannot be brought back to normal, even though they may be improved. The duration of the cure is proportional to the degree of the deficiency.

Detoxification symptoms are often considered reactions by the uninformed. These symptoms develop when more toxins are liberated from the system than can be eliminated by the body. With good elimination there are few detoxification symptoms. Since detoxification is an essential part of the process of getting well nutritionally, there must be good doctor-patient cooperation and understanding of the process taking place.

Sometimes one gland is restored to health more rapidly than other organs. This can and does create peculiar symptoms, which might be thoughtlessly blamed on the program. In such a case, the simplest and most effective course is to discontinue therapy for a short time, followed by resumption after the symptoms subside. If this fails again, the program should be altered or revised downward to fit the individual needs. Every patient is different and unique in his particular needs.

Lack of Response

Assuming that the patient is following the program as directed, there are some reasons why the nutritional program may not be working. One is insufficient dosage. Not enough nutrients are being used to accomplish the mission. Another obvious area is insufficient time. It takes real time for the body to eliminate toxins and to rebuild normal tissue and metabolic response. I nearly gave up on one woman, who then suddenly normalized after eighteen weeks on the nutritional program. It was very discouraging at first, but the finale was beautiful.

Response of the various organs differs greatly. Nerve tissue takes much longer to rebuild than other tissues. Patient needs vary. All heart cases do not respond in the same way. Each has his own manner and degree of response. Every patient is unique.

CHAPTER VI

HYPOGLYCEMIA: A COMMON DENOMINATOR

RECENTLY A QUESTION reached me through my column in *Let's Live Magazine*. This is a pathetic story of a woman who was looking for help for an ailment that she had learned to diagnose for herself: low blood sugar, known by the medical term, hypoglycemia. This woman had not received any help or diagnosis elsewhere but had read widely, searching for light on her problem. She never received it. She is not an exception; she is the rule in this country today. Because it is a "new disease," not been taught in medical school, 99 percent of doctors do not recognize it, let alone treat it properly. To let the woman speak for herself:

"I have suffered from low blood sugar or hypoglycemia, as I now know the correct name, most of my life. Sometimes there would be a year or more without a blackout. As I grew older, they became more severe and harder to recover from until, finally, I was constantly sick. Doctors just did not know what was wrong with me. Most of them said I just suffered from complete exhaustion due to overwork. I did not believe them, because it was obviously not true. Very few believed what I said; they always made me feel that I had an overactive imagination and they refused to be concerned.

"Finally a friend sent me to a health store where I found the book *Body, Mind and Sugar** by E.M. Abra-

*Pyramid Publications, New York, N.Y. Paperback. 1971.

hamson, M.D. After reading the book I was sure I had found out what was wrong with me, so I called the School of Medicine in the large and famous university near me. I told the doctors I had found my trouble and asked if they would take me. They finally agreed. When I went, they turned me over to an internist. I asked for a glucose tolerance test which was stated in the Abrahamson book as a *must* for detecting hypoglycemia. The internist said this was not my trouble but he finally agreed to give me one anyway. After the test they sent me to the endocrinology clinic. After several months of tests they told me not to come back. When I asked the doctors if they could help me, they said, 'No, you have too many complications.'

"Since then, I have tried many physicians, with little help. I have had to work out a diet for myself but it is not complete because I have such terrible reactions such as violent muscle spasms in the stomach area, and sleeplessness which makes me feel as if I am high on dope and I feel so wound up. Few foods agree with me. If I eat salt, I wake up in the night with my tongue stuck tight to the roof of my mouth. Any medication starts a reaction and I swell up, turn red and feel as if I am going to have a heart attack; it is so hard to breathe. I am tired all the time and shaky much of the time.

"I heard of the Hypoglycemia Foundation and wrote them a letter. All they did was to send me some literature and ask for money. They did not tell me anything in the literature I didn't already know. Since then, I have been from doctor to doctor. In most cases, they don't even seem to want to try to help me. I am really desperate and disillusioned."

Despair of Patients

Frequently, when patients like this come to me, when they finally reach me, they are at their wit's end. They usually say that if I cannot help them, they will give up trying to find help. Fortunately, my approach helps most of them. It is true that I neither blame such patients for their overactive imagination, nor give them a tranquilizer or a pep pill to get rid of them, nor turn them away. In the beginning, I was actually forced by my conscience and by my patients to find out what was wrong with them. The result was my becoming a specialist in hypoglycemia. I was amazed to find that this disturbance, low blood sugar, was a common denominator, not only among countless patients but also in many other ailments. When it was corrected other health problems also vanished.

The History of Hypoglycemia

The condition popularly known as hypoglycemia is a very controversial subject in medical circles today. There is no agreement on definition of the term. It has been known since the discovery of insulin in the early twenties. Seale Harris, M.D. was the first one to popularize the concept of diet as a causative factor. He was followed by Hans Selye, M.D. who postulated the stress-adaption syndrome. Later, John Tintera, M.D. put these factors into practical terms; he used a dietary approach combined with the injection of adrenocortical extract (ACE) as therapeutic measures.

The press has actually popularized the concept of hypoglycemia. The newspapers are printing more articles on the subject; there are features in magazines. The general awakening to ecology has made people more aware of their own bodies in relation to improved nutrition. Proof is worshiped, theory is scorned by so-called experts. Hypoglycemia has been a "theoretical" stepchild no doctor is anxious to adopt.

The doctors are nevertheless being made aware of hypoglycemia by their patients. Many patients have read articles on hypoglycemia and have seen themselves described. They, naturally, go to their own doctors to discuss their new-found suspicions. Doctors react in various manners. Some say, "I am your doctor and know what to do for you. I may not know what is wrong with you, but I do know what you do not have." Some cooperate and order the glucose tolerance test as requested but fail in the interpretations. Others refuse outright to order the test.

Education

Education is the only way to get people and doctors to know the complete story of hypoglycemia. The facts are simple and easy to understand and believe when taught properly. There is also a great need for a variety of good, naturally grown, fresh and raw food to feed these patients. Physicians and patients should be seriously trained in nutrition. Except for stress, nutrition is the only major causal factor in the disease which can be controlled. Thus, it should be the primary target in all areas of therapeutics. Hypoglycemia is no exception. The body reacts to food according to the kind of food provided. It is a form of fuel. High-quality fuel promotes better health. Foodless foods do not promote health.

Hypoglycemics are not even being nutritionally helped in hospitals, where the dietary is an example of the worst type. If there is anything that is furthest from a natural and organic approach, it is hospital fare. Foods are overcooked, steamed, and loaded with sugar and man-made carbohydrates. In many homes the diet is not much better. No wonder health is declining in this country.

Because of patient pressure, organized medicine is beginning to say the words used in hypoglycemic circles, without understanding what they mean. They prefer to pass the buck to a specialist, who may know more than the GP does. For instance, one writer has listed ten types of hypoglycemia. Nine of these require the assistance of a psychiatrist. The tenth, they claim, needs a surgeon. This whole maneuver, of course, removes the burden of trying to understand the patient from the doctor's shoulders and protects the status quo of the medical profession.

Symptoms of Hypoglycemia

Some common symptoms experienced by hypoglycemics include the following:

General

cold sweats	anxiety
convulsions	tremulousness or shakiness
fainting or blackout spells	fearfulness
"going crazy" sensation	claustrophobia
emotional upsets	numbness or pain sensation
unstable temper	weakness
moody	craving for sweets
sleepy after meals	faintness if meals delayed
stuffy nose	irritability
fatigue	sleepiness, especially in daytime
exhaustion	and after meals
confusion	edema
can't think straight	can't decide easily

Gastrointestinal

indigestion	colitis
gas	diarrhea

flatus (abdominal gas)	bloating
abdominal pain	itching anus
ulcer syndrome	

Eye, Ear, Nose, Throat

blurred vision	hoarseness
tinnitus	dizziness
peculiar tastes or smells	dry mouth

Cardiorespiratory

arrhythmias	shortness of breath
pain	

Genitourinary

menstrual problems	loss of libido
sexual behavior deviations	burning on urination
frequency of urination	

Skin

bronzing tendency	thin, clammy

Bone, Joint, Muscle

arthritic tendencies	twitching of eyelids
burning feet	cold extremities

These disease syndromes (symptoms) can sometimes be caused by hypoglycemia:

anxiety states	allergic states
schizophrenia	abnormal sexual behavior
ulcer	alcoholism
colitis	arthritic syndromes

Hypoglycemics feel better temporarily after:

eating sweets	drinking alcohol or smoking
drinking coffee	cigarettes

Fortunately, there are some early signs of acceptance of the concept of hypoglycemia found in my own practice. At first, the regular medical men insisted that the disturbance did not exist. As time went on they saw that the problem did not go away. They then said, "It does exist, but it is misdiagnosed." They again implied that treatment should be handled by a surgeon or a psychiatrist. Later they admitted, "It does exist but is grossly overtreated." Currently they are saying, "It does exist, but go somewhere else for treatment." Since their "problem" still will not go away, I wonder what the next tactic will be.

There are also many cases of misdiagnosis in patients who have been erroneously admitted to mental hospitals when their true condition was merely hypoglycemia—a fact discovered upon their release.

My definition for hypoglycemia is that it is an abnormal glucose (sugar) metabolism, evidenced by persistently low or insufficient rise in blood sugar after eating or drinking carbohydrates and/or sudden, profound or precipitous drops in blood sugar in immediate or delayed response to eating sugar. NOTE: Natural carbohydrates and starches do not cause hypoglycemia, but once it is established, they can and do perpetuate it. Man-made carbohydrates, such as refined white sugar and white flour, complicated by stress, are the main causes of hypoglycemia.

I find hypoglycemia a common condition in my practice. In fact, I assume it to be present until proven otherwise.

Theory of Hypoglycemia

Hypoglycemia is caused by hyperinsulinism. There are two major mechanisms for the production of too much insulin. In the first type there is an overproduction of insulin by the beta cells of the pancreas. This, in my estimation, is caused by repeated ingestion of processed carbohydrates. The situation develops like this: whenever the blood sugar rises, the pancreas "feels" the need for insulin so it produces insulin and puts it into the blood. The insulin-sugar reaction takes place and the sugar level is lowered. This pancreatic mechanism normally occurs at the beginning of a meal or whenever food or beverage is taken. The rub comes when processed carbohydrates are consumed and the pancreas responds as if a big meal were about to be consumed. The pancreas reacts as it should normally, except now the situation is not normal. Instead of a normal meal expected by the pancreas, the food eaten is probably a carbohydrate or a sugar product, such as a Danish, a donut, some candy, cake or ice cream. Suddenly, there is more insulin produced than needed and the sugar level plummets downward toward subnormal levels. The person feels weak, shaky, tired or cross. He may even black out. This routine is repeated, more or less, every time man-made carbohydrates are eaten. It is also repeated with every cup of coffee drunk or cigarette smoked. Day in and day out, weeks extend into months and years. The blood sugar rises *temporarily,* but what goes up must come down. The reaction mechanism gets more and more delicately unbalanced. In time, the pancreas begins to react to other types of circumstances such as fear or anger. The adrenalin secreted by the adrenal medulla causes the liver to send more glucose into the blood which then causes the pancreas to overreact in insulin production. Ultimately, we have a mechanism which has gone completely out of control. Hyperinsulinism can now be triggered at the drop of a hat.

It has been generally accepted according to usual knowledge that diabetes is the opposite of hypoglycemia as far as blood sugar activity is concerned.

There are other, rare pancreatic conditions causing hypoglycemia, such as tumors of the beta cells, but the one I have described is by far the most common.

Anti-Insulin

The balancing force to the production of insulin by the pancreas is the production of the anti-insulin factors by the adrenal cortex. This second major theory of hyperinsulinism is the extension of the Hans Selye, M.D. concept also popularized by John Tintera, M.D. Their theory is that the adrenal cortex glands become exhausted by excessive stress. This, in turn, curtails natural body production of anti-insulin factors with resultant hyperinsulinism and hypoglycemia.

Stress

Types of stress can be physical, emotional, chemical, and nutritional. Physical stress is merely overwork with insufficient rest. Emotional stress needs no definition. Everyone has it. Chemical stress is an ecological, integral part of our lives. Poisons via food, air and water are getting into our bodies. They do not belong there. Since they are abnormal elements in the body, they must be eliminated by the body. We cannot escape the chemicals in our environment, but nutritional stress can be controlled, and this is one thing I can teach the patient to do. If he can control physical and nutritional stress, his body can be strengthened to better resist the inroads of environmental stress. Failure to control all four stresses spells disaster. Stresses overwork the adrenal cortex glands. The adrenal cortex glands are the antistress centers. Thus, if we are exposed to too much stress, the cortex becomes exhausted. We are not talking about total exhaustion, called Addison's disease, at this point, but merely a partial or subclinical exhaustion. Some function persists but it is insufficient for adrenocortical adequate performances. The result is insufficient anti-insulin factors being secreted into the blood, resulting in hyper-insulinism and hypoglycemia.

It is also quite apparent that the causative factors of hypoglycemia are not limited to the pancreas and adrenal cortex. The pituitary gland is intimately involved. Pituitary failure can result in adrenocortical failure. The liver cannot be ignored either, since it is the storehouse for glycogen, the chemical form of sugar, which is converted into blood glucose as a result of demand by adrenalin. Harmony among all the endocrine glands is a must before good health can exist.

There is one fairly common finding in glucose tolerance test results: blood sugar levels are frequently very high during the first two or three hours, only to fall to great depths later. Such patients appear to be diabetics in the early part of the test but are hypoglycemic in the latter part. I call this reaction "dysinsulinism." In my experience, treatment for dysinsulinism is the same as that for hypoglycemia. *Dysinsulinism cannot be diagnosed without the aid of the five-hour glucose tolerance test.* If only the three-hour test is used, these patients could and are being misdiagnosed as diabetic! A misdiagnosis leads to a therapeutic program aimed in the wrong direction. This can be a very difficult patient to manage, to say the least.

CHAPTER VII

SOME CASE HISTORIES

HERE ARE a few case histories of patients who have had their health improved through nutritional therapy. Most of these patients felt hopeless and never expected to enjoy good health again.

You can see by their testimonies, written in their own words, the remarkable changes which nutritional therapy accomplished for them.

CASE HISTORY: Hypoglycemia

"Since 1955 I have attempted to convince twenty-three physicians that I was ill. Along with being insulted and accused of being psychosomatic and paranoid, I was given tranquilizers and hormones, none of which helped.

"I was suffering from exhaustion, fainting spells, emotional upsets, confusion, shaky limbs, weakness, dizziness, palpitations, arthritic tendencies and a constant feeling of extreme heat.

"Approximately five years ago I tried to convince some of these physicians that I believed that I had low blood sugar and I was further insulted and called a food faddist because I was attempting to control my condition through better nutrition, consisting of natural foods and vitamin supplements.

"Three years ago I met a woman who told me about Dr. Nittler's work. Shortly thereafter I consulted Dr. Nittler and after careful examination and numerous laboratory tests he confirmed my suspected diagnosis of hypoglycemia. For two years and a half I have been on his program of natural foods, vitamin supplements and injections.

"Because my condition had been neglected by previous physicians, I was very ill and my entire body was not functioning properly. During the past two years I have improved enormously under Dr. Nittler's treatment and am now able to function more normally. I am convinced that a continuance of Dr. Nittler's program for another year or two will bring even further improvement."

CASE HISTORY: Hypoglycemia

"I am a 45-year-old housewife. About nine months ago I became very ill with flu. I was too ill to go to a doctor and as I did not have a fever, I knew there was no need to have a doctor come to the house. After two weeks I was no better and still had such extreme weakness I needed help to get to the bathroom and even had trouble feeding myself. I called our doctor and was told flu was bad this year and I'd just have to fight it out. Headache was a very predominant complaint.

"After three weeks with no improvement, my husband took me to a doctor. The effort of walking about a hundred feet from the car to the doctor's office caused my heart to start fibrillating. I was immediately sent next door to see an internist, who did a cardiogram and a blood analysis. They then told me I had a severe case of virus flu and all I could do was wait for it to leave. Of course, this was very discouraging, as I was sure I could not be so sick from flu only after all this time.

"A friend from out of town eventually heard about my illness and called me and asked me to call Dr. Nittler. After five weeks in bed, I was still too weak to even care for myself, so I was happy to hear of a doctor who might be able to help me. I made an appointment with Dr. Nittler the next day. After the reports of various tests were returned, Dr. Nittler told me I had hypoglycemia. I went on Dr. Nittler's recommended diet and food supplements, and gradually started to regain my strength.

"For four or five years prior to getting flu, I had been having problems with nervousness, anxiety, weight loss, dizziness, heart flutters, palpitations and pain, an inability to concentrate and almost daily headaches which were frequently severe and accompanied by nausea. At that time I was told that although my cardiogram was not normal, my heart was fine and the deviation and heart noises were caused by something outside the heart. Except for being underweight and a borderline diabetic, I was pronounced to be in excellent health.

"All of my problems have subsided or disappeared since being under Dr. Nittler's care. I rarely have a headache now, which is a great blessing to me as I had really been tormented by them. I've gained back the weight I lost and added a few more needed pounds. I'm able to care for my family and home again, and every month I can see gains toward better health than I've known for years."

CASE HISTORY: Hypoglycemia

"I have been in poor health most of my life, and my trouble has been diagnosed as various things, including a low-grade virus infection, constitutional inadequacy, and the menopause.

"When I was about twenty-two years old (about thirty-five years ago), I had vague symptoms of fatigue, back pains and nervousness and after going to several doctors, I consulted a gynecologist who prescribed hormones. They didn't seem to help much but I took them for years and gradually had to add sedatives in order to sleep. But each sleeping pill (phenobarbital, seconal) soon lost its effectiveness and I still couldn't sleep. I felt as though my whole body was very tense day and night, and it seemed to me there must be something in my system that was keeping me awake. All the usual suggestions for curing insomnia did not work.

"Finally, when I was about forty years old, I had a long illness in which I felt weak and tired but had no severe symptoms. However, I had to take a seven months leave of absence from my job, and after an exploratory operation which revealed nothing, I was advised to take a complete rest. I went to Arizona for three months, but it didn't help much. I was eventually able to go back to work, but I could do nothing but that for about three years.

"I had a physical examination every year and was always told that I was fine. Then why did I feel so miserable? I was given tranquilizers to help me sleep and I took aspirin by the bottle just to keep going.

"This went on for several years, and every winter I would have a long siege of the flu which kept me from my job four or five weeks. I often felt much better by evening, and would tell the office that I would be back to work in the morning, but by morning I felt worse and couldn't go.

"I finally decided to retire and in my leisure time indulged in more sweets such as ice cream and lemonade. Before that my diet had been fairly good, with very few sweets and starches although I did find myself eating Lifesavers often on the job. After retirement, I began to feel worse and worse. Finally a new doctor gave me a five-hour glucose tolerance test which showed that I had low blood sugar. He suggested that I eat a high-protein diet about six times a day and skip the sugar. This helped and at times I felt wonderful, better than I ever had in my life. But it didn't last and I began to feel worse and worse.

"It was then that I heard about Dr. Nittler and sought his help. After about two months of intensive treatment I began to improve and, although I still have my ups and downs, I feel that I am on the right track. I am now sleeping well without tranquilizers or sleeping pills for the first time in years. My energy is much improved and I am beginning to be able to think again."

CASE HISTORY: Kidney Stones

"During the first week in May 1960 I had my first experience with kidney stones. While returning from a fishing trip and enjoying apparent good health, I suddenly was taken with a severe pain in the left side midway between the lower rib and my groin. While staying overnight in a hospital, I passed a small stone which the doctor stated was a uric acid crystal.

"About nineteen years ago I had an accident going over a 13-foot ledge on horseback, with the horse rolling over me twice. I had no apparent serious injury at the time; however, six months later both knees and ankles became intensely painful and then swelled considerably. This condition became chronic, recurring every six or eight months, sometimes to such an extent I would be on crutches or even a wheelchair for several weeks at a time.

"Approximately twelve years ago, 1959, I learned I could successfully control this apparent lodging of the uric acid in my tendons and tendon sheaths by taking one antiuric acid tablet in the evening and one in the morning.

"While on another hunting trip in October 1969, I had my second severe kidney stone attack. After nineteen hours of intense pain I successfully passed some "uric acid gravel." A doctor advised me to keep some bladder sedative tablets handy in case of a future attack. He claimed these would anesthetize the urinary tract and help somewhat in passing a stone.

"During the first six months of 1971, I passed small stones on four separate occasions, each time within eight hours of the first sign of pain. Only once did I use the tablets prescribed by the doctor.

"Upon consulting with my physician, Dr. Alan Nittler, I was cautioned that it was very possible I could have an attack and the stone might be too large to pass.

"On July 22, 1971, while driving from my home, I had another attack. This time the pain would last a few hours then abate sometimes for a complete day or so. This condition continued with the attacks becoming more severe with accompanying headache, backache, constipation, nausea, etc. All the time I drank all the water I could hold. On August 18, Dr. Nittler recommended I take two magnesium oxide tablets (250 mg. each) per day. On August 23 about 8:30 P.M. I started passing what appeared to be small pieces of bloody tissue. At 10:30 P.M. I finally passed a large stone, measuring 7/16" long and 3/16" diameter.

"I am positive the magnesium oxide tablets made it possible to pass this large stone which had been causing pain for over thirty days. I am also very grateful that Dr. Nittler persuaded me to 'hang on for a few more days,' continuing the treatment. My only alternative was an operation."

CASE HISTORY: "The Pill"

"I am eighteen years old and attend college. I had never had a menstrual period and our family doctor felt nothing needed to be done about it. I was quite well developed by the time I was twelve and had expected it for some time. When I was nearly fifteen, I went to a gynecologist who put me on The Pill. While on The Pill I did have regular periods, with cramps; but when I was taken off The Pill the periods stopped. As I did not want to take The Pill anymore, I had not had a period for over a year when I first went to Dr. Nittler. After three months on Dr. Nittler's prescribed diet and food supplements I had a period with no complications and have had monthly periods for over a year. A severe acne problem I've had since fifth grade (eight years) has improved considerably and has almost disappeared. Many months of visits to a dermatologist when I was twelve and thirteen had made no improvement in my skin problem."

CASE HISTORY: Pregnancy

"To start with I ruined my health while going to college. Later, while working and being a new homemaker, my diet was still far from acceptable. Also, at work I was exposed to a very great deal of ammonia fumes while working with blueprints. When I became pregnant I was worried and decided things must change. I sought—and received—nutritional help.

"I began taking numerous food supplements routinely. For the second through the fifth months I was on a strict diet excluding meat. This was done because of the presence of albumin in my urine. The sixth to ninth months were albumin free and I maintained a very well balanced diet.

"My baby arrived, a very healthy and beautiful little girl without any complications and with ease of delivery. I tried to nurse her, but, due to the excitement involved with my husband's return home from Navy duty, it was impossible. We fed her a mixture of milk, water and honey. At about 2 weeks we started her on whole grain brown rice which was ground and cooked then mixed with honey and milk. At about 2-1/2 weeks we began feeding her crushed avocado. Gradually we increased the variety of her foods to include fresh vegetables and fruits which I pureed myself. At 6 months she decided she was going to eat table food and has since then.

"She was a discontented child, until 1 year, when she walked, not because she was unhealthy but because she was always mentally ready to do things her body couldn't. For example, at 3 days she was able to lift her head and hold it up. She is now 19 months old and says four-word sentences quite often and is constantly babbling sentences of two or three words. She can say any word except maybe antidisestablishmentarianism. She knows her full name. She can even count a little and knows colors. Her coordination and balance are better than mine and she knows everything that is going on and some of the contemplated results. She is a well-balanced child.

"I am now pregnant again and am doing much the same as with my girl. We know our next one will be as healthy mentally, physically and spiritually."

CASE HISTORY: Heart Attack

"From the experiences I've had the past several years, I'm confident I had suffered several 'silent heart attacks' prior to my first coronary in June 1968 at the age of forty-six. During several particularly stressful periods I now realize the distress and discomfort I experienced on two very vivid occasions were similar, except for intensity, to the pains I experienced in June 1968.

"Following usual medical attention, which included two weeks in Coronary Care Unit at our local hospital, plus two weeks' additional hospitalization, I progressed gradually through a five-month period of increased activity. Our family physician had been summoned by a registered nurse neighbor, who quickly observed the typical signs of a coronary: profuse sweating, vomiting and (in my case) acute pains across the shoulders. During the five months of inactivity, I was started on a walking program progressing from 5 minutes in the morning and 5 minutes in the afternoon to a total of 2 hours a day; then bicycling. After ten months, all medication was eliminated and the salt-free diet discontinued. I was encouraged to continue on a low-fat diet which had been my diet pattern for the previous eight years. I was encouraged to keep my weight at 150 lbs. which was 15 lbs. less than when the coronary occurred.

"I can honestly say I felt good and was convinced I had readjusted my life pattern and had learned to pace myself to be more free of self-imposed pressures. I had been led to believe that job pressures, including tight schedules and many projects all going at once, were as much responsible for my health problems as anything else.

"However, on Easter Sunday, March 29, 1970, I suffered not only another occlusion, but an acute cardiac arrest. This was preceded by three days of intense weariness, fatigue and restlessness during which time our same family physician counseled: 'Stay home, rest and do nothing.' Unfortunately, he was out of town from the time he was first called until the day following the cardiac arrest. Only extreme good fortune or luck made it possible for me to write these words. The same registered nurse neighbor who was called during my first attack was again available. She would have been gone on a family picnic ten minutes later. She administered mouth-to-mouth resuscitation while our teenage son performed chest massage under her direction. The arrival of the ambulance brought another registered nurse neighbor, who works in the emergency room of our hospital, and her husband who is in charge of the X-ray unit at the same hospital. Together they continued the mouth-to-mouth resuscitation and chest massage during the ambulance trip to the hospital. I understand a number of 400-volt electric shock treatments were required to reestablish a regular heart beat. I was unconscious for a number of hours and do not recall events for a five-day period following the attack and events of the preceding three days are extremely hazy.

"One week in Coronary Care and two weeks' hospitalization brought me home again. Within 2-1/2 months our family doctor counseled a cardiac reserve test at a nearby metropolitan area medical center. He was advised by their personnel to take me off all medication for ten days prior to the scheduled tests. Upon arrival at the medical center, my pulse was 104 and the doctors expressed deep concern over fluid buildup in my lungs and liver.

"Needless to say, no tests could be conducted and they immediately began to make arrangements for me to undergo catheter tests which, I understand, requires tubes up through veins in the arms into the chambers of the heart to pinpoint where the trouble is and help determine if open heart surgery can correct the problem. They hoped this would be the case, at least, for they believed open heart surgery to be the only hope for giving me a normal life span. Our family doctor immediately prescribed up to 6 digitalis tablets a day until the fluid subsided. My chart stated that I once again had experienced congestive heart failure.

"It was at this point that I was referred to Dr. Nittler. I need not describe his method of treating me. Suffice it to say, after his initial examination and after reviewing my medical history, including all X-rays, etc. made available to him, he started me on his 'basic heart program.' On August 3, 1970, I started on his complete detoxification program, etc. Within weeks, I noticed great improvement. By late September, I felt an increased surge of well-being with each passing week. My family doctor continues to monitor my case. He cannot, at this point, rule out the open heart surgery recommended by his peers, but he is honest enough to admit that I've shown great improvement. He says my heart is beating more slowly and stronger and that everything sounds good. My laboratory tests are all normal, including a cholesterol count of 189. These tests were made in November. Dr. Nittler says in his judgment I can rule out open heart surgery to which I most heartily agree. My local doctor still has me on disability but I'm looking forward to returning to work and a normal productive life."

CASE HISTORY: Asthma

"I've been subject to asthma all my life. It would come with a cold or when I laughed or exercised too hard. The situation became dramatically worse when we moved to Santa Cruz in 1966. For some reason I'd catch a cold every four to six weeks. I had a brand-new baby and we just seemed to pass the cold back and forth. Only when I got it, it would go into my chest, develop into asthma and I could hardly breathe. I was fed up with being sick and tired all the time but was not ready to take advantage of Dr. Nittler's help. I was very ignorant and prejudiced against his nutritional approach. I had to be driven to desperation before I became his patient. One night in 1968 I sat up all night with asthma (just from a *cold)*, the medicine I'd taken was not helping at all. I finally became so desperate I had to awaken the whole family and have my husband drive me to the hospital at about 4:00 A.M. for a shot to relieve my difficult breathing.

"So I went through Dr. Nittler's whole program and learned a lot about nutrition and health and eating as the months went by. The first dramatic proof I had that the program was really working for me was about six months after I started it. We were with some good friends and everyone was letting down their hair. We laughed and laughed at silly jokes and games. All of a sudden it struck me that I *should* have been choked up and gasping for breath because of asthma—but I wasn't—not a hint of it! Now (1971) the few colds I catch are very mild. I can't even remember the last time I had asthma with or without a cold!"

CASE HISTORY: Poor Health

"This is the true story of one of the many patients of Dr. Alan Nittler, and I can offer help to those of you, who, like myself have managed to survive more than fifty years. First off, the age of nine was the beginning of a life of multiple surgeries and under the constant care of the medical profession. I was constantly told that, just because I had the desire and wanted to do the many things that others do, I must never try to compete and must take life easy. Then, to make life more complicated, ten years ago I was in an auto accident and as a result was left housebound. I had had three bone fusions and many months of hospitalization, under constant pain and given an unlimited supply of narcotics. All of the consulting doctors merely said that they wished they could do more for me and gave me unlimited prescriptions. Then, perchance, while confined to home, unable to ride in an auto for more than fifty miles and totally incapable of driving, I read about Dr. Nittler. I felt a ray of hope and so I asked my husband if I could consult him, promising that this would be the last doctor I would consult. No one can possibly imagine the joy I have experienced. After being with Dr. Nittler for ten months, I was capable of driving 4,000 miles on a vacation. The sheer joy of just seeing nature, walking beaches, gathering all sorts of rock, driftwood and conversing with people is more than I can convey. Not one soul suspected that I was not perfect. Now, let me warn all who seek Dr. Nittler's help. His program is stiff and for months I was discouraged and thought that I should improve faster, then I would ask myself if it took years for me to get into this shape, how could I expect to recover faster? But I am recovering! My family cannot believe the change in me and, while I am not perfect, I am now able to work forty hours per week, keep house, tend a small garden and pursue hobbies. So, I say to all, there is hope."

CASE HISTORY: Diabetes; Stroke
(as reported by a patient's wife)

"In February 1961 my husband, who was then 64, felt completely well except for some minor arthritic pains, some slight bloating and gas disturbances, and occasionally a charley horse in his legs or thighs. He was an avid gardener.

"We had been married about a year when, at my urging, he went for a complete medical check (the first in forty years). The doctor diagnosed diabetes. At that time he weighed about 190 pounds. To hold the diabetes in control, he was given 250 mg. of a hypoglycemic agent to take daily and he was put on a 1300-calorie diet. He gave away the home-canned jellies I'd made and stopped the nightly wedge of pie with ice cream, but he still ate enormous amounts of canned and fresh fruits and cereals and bread, plus reasonably heavy meals which he cooked himself (I was working). He just totally ignored the 1300-calorie diet he was supposed to follow, and put dietetic jelly on everything. He did all the housework and still gardened avidly.

"I quit work and took over the household duties. My husband still gardened, but I could see he was visibly slowed down. He refused to travel any distance from home because he had stiffness in his whole body, especially in his legs—his charley horse bothered him. He began to complain a lot more of gas, and also that he had a burning sensation when urinating.

"He was now being checked by the doctor every three months. The doctor discovered a heart irregularity and my husband was given three tablets of Quinidine four times daily to steady his heartbeat, and also a hypoglycemic agent.

"Almost immediately, he had a light stroke. As a result, his left arm was affected and he had no grip when he tried to grasp any object; his left leg dragged slightly when he walked. He wasn't able to talk, although he could make sounds. He overcame the worst of the stroke but he always seemed to be exhausted, and slept a lot, day and night. He looked terrible—poor skin color, with a wizened, anxious expression on his face all the time. When he got up from a chair, I could see it was a great physical effort for him. By exercising his left leg and arm, eventually he got to the point where he was able to walk one short block. His speech got better, but it was still somewhat garbled. He still had some physical complaints.

"He picked up and read FDA, AMA and American Diabetes Association Reports which say the hypoglycemic agent caused heart derangements, and when he pointed these out to me I said he should see another doctor. We went to our local health food store and asked if they knew of any physician who treated patients in nature's way, sans medication. The clerk supplied a couple of names, but my husband refused to travel several hundred miles to any of these doctors. The clerk then suggested a local chiropractor, and my husband went to see this man, who emphatically advised him to get treatment from Dr. Nittler. My husband was feeling miserable, and he finally made an appointment for November 1970.

"Dr. Nittler's therapy started. A complete examination disclosed not only diabetes, but also hypoglycemia, a combination diagnosis known as dysinsulinism. The doctor gave him massive doses of selected vitamins, plus nutritional injections. Almost immediately I could see my husband perk up; his skin color improved and his old enthusiasms were back. His weight was down to 175 pounds.

"He now says he feels much better. He can walk a mile easily, his foot doesn't drag anymore, and he doesn't complain about aches and pains. He can grasp objects and do simple chores around the house. He's gone back to gardening the way he did when we were first married, and he doesn't nap in the daytime.

"Under Dr. Nittler's care he gradually cut down on

both medications and finally could discontinue them entirely.

"He's learned to use the diabetic test tape four times a day, and it's let him discover for himself which foods are safe for him and which to avoid. Dr. Nittler says this is all-important, and this eating the safe foods plus continuing the vitamin therapy should add many healthful years to my husband's life. I'm delighted."

CASE HISTORY: Skin disease with Physical Complications

"What a pleasure it is to meet and know Dr. Alan H. Nittler, M.D., while, at the same time, having him help your health to improve beyond your highest hopes within a period of eight weeks.

"Prior to meeting Dr. Nittler, my wife and I thought we were pretty nutrition conscious. In fact, we had to be. For through the use of prednisone to control my lupus erythematosus, I'd developed some unhappy side effects: diabetic tendencies and a heart problem. With these you are forced to diet.

"In the beginning your confidence builds when Dr. Nittler gives you a battery of physical and functional tests. Then, after the total analyses, he spends an hour explaining the results of your physical examination, even letting you take home a group of punch cards from the laboratory tests for your files.

"But even more impressive is getting down to business with the basic detoxification program and wonderful vitamin and food supplements that do so many things for your physical and mental well-being.

"Both of us, after the first eight weeks, feel the results were phenomenal and we never want to go back to old food or eating habits.

"In my case, an allopathic, sophisticated internist had been keeping me going with 15 mg. of prednisone a day, a hypoglycemic agent for the diabetes, and digitalis for the heart. The internist, an empathetic man and well intentioned, knew and talked about the side effects of so much prednisone. But he offered no solution.

"Thanks to Dr. Nittler, I have stopped taking the latter medication and have cut the amount of prednisone from 15 mg. to between 2-1/2 and 5 mg. All this in only eight weeks after years of medication.

"Beyond the treatments however is the stimulating experience of knowing Dr. Nittler. He is a dedicated, devoutly religious man and sparkles with enthusiasm over organic avocados he raises, the fertile eggs his chickens lay, and many other interesting things.

"My wife and I feel what this country needs is at least a thousand Dr. Nittlers, nutritionally oriented, to offset the terrible damage drugs and processed foods are doing to people."

CASE HISTORY: Ulcer Syndrome

"When I first went to the doctor, my stomach was bothering me, terribly. After examinations, the doctor discovered I had ulcers. The doctor that I was then going to gave me pills and antacids to kill the pain.

"My father was dissatisfied with what my doctor was doing for me. He had heard of a nutritional doctor, Dr. Nittler, and thought he could be of more help to me. As soon as possible, we made an appointment to go to Dr. Nittler. When I went to him, he took my father and me into his office and we told him the problem. The doctor was willing to help us.

"The doctor made an appointment for me to come back a week later for tests. After the completion of the tests, the doctor had found I had hypoglycemia (which means 'below normal blood sugar'). My doctor explained to my family that it wasn't just the ulcer, but the cause behind it, which complicated the problem.

"From the result of his findings, he put me on a diet, gave me special pills, and gave me shots of ACE.

"A month after I had been going to Dr. Nittler, I went back to my first doctor. He was surprised to find that my ulcer had improved a lot, and that I was feeling much better. When I first started with Dr. Nittler, I felt fine, I thought; but now I have a lot more energy. I do a lot more things, and I really like to live now."

CASE HISTORY: Dysinsulinism

"In April of the year 1970, I came to Dr. Nittler, after eight years of unsuccessful treatment to relieve my symptoms.

"At the age of twenty-nine I had a hysterectomy; a year after this operation my health began to fail. I was extremely tired, no pep or energy. I was very tense—even though things in my life were going well, I still had, and could get no relief from it. I would wake up in the middle of the night and could not get back to sleep. I felt blue and depressed even when my surroundings were cheerful. I lost my sense of well-being.

"I was not successful in taking hormone replacement for this; I was found to be sensitive to therapy.

"When I came to Dr. Nittler he ran a series of tests so that he could get a complete picture of the whole body. In doing this he found along with my hormone deficiency other conditions contributing to my symptoms. He found I had a condition known as dysinsulinism and was not assimilating my proteins properly, and my fat metabolism was also inadequate. He found my heart had to work harder to do a normal task.

"He set up a complete program to help the whole body and, after six months of this treatment, I am feeling much better, in fact better than I have in eight years. I believe that with continuation of this program in the future I will be symptom free."

CASE HISTORY: Allergic Hives

"In the latter part of last November, I broke out in an allergic dermatitis — severe hives. My first visit to my regular family doctor was a couple of days later. I was given medication to take at home. A few days after this, with no helpful effects, the medication was changed. Again, a few days of treatment proved futile; my condition became worse. In addition to the hives, I would get a severe pain in an area above the right kidney, but rather centrally located. This pain would come and go, lasting from five minutes to one hour. It was an acute shattering pain that immobilized me. I was next given cortisone. After twenty-four hours this would lessen the severity of both hives and pain. As long as I continued with cortisone (for four or five days each time) I was fine, but when I stopped, severe hives and pain reoccurred. Then back to cortisone four or five days, followed by severe hives and pain. I seesawed back and forth in this manner for about seven weeks. Finally I was told that the cortisone should be discontinued and my next move was to go to a university medical center hospital.

"A friend of mine gave me Dr. Alan H. Nittler's telephone number and begged me to call him immediately, since he was the only person who had helped his son afflicted with a severe ailment. This young man had visited two major medical centers before he visited Dr. Nittler.

"The father of this young man was so insistent that I call Dr. Nittler (he even offered to assist financially with the new medical expense, if I would go to Dr. Nittler—though I did not accept) that I did so, but not without a little misgiving and apprehension on my part because I did not think help was coming my way.

"Dr. Nittler asked me to come in the next morning, January 16, 1970. I was put on a limited diet immediately supplemented with various vitamins. In the course of the days to follow, I was without cortisone. This permitted the dread hives and pain to expose themselves!

"Then on the tenth day under Dr. Nittler's care, something wonderful (to me, a miracle) happened— I was *free* of my ailments! A staggering weight had been lifted from both my shoulders and my wife's. She had been so concerned and worried, I thought she would have a nervous breakdown. Now, as I am in the thirteenth month under the doctor's care, I am enjoying the best of health and feeling great."

CASE HISTORY: Lupus Erythematosus

"When Judi was thirteen years old and in the eighth grade, her fingers began to get swollen and stiff. Also, her jaws were sore and kept popping. She couldn't open her mouth wide enough to get around an apple. Her periods became irregular. During the summer we went on a long trip and by the time we got back, all of her joints were stiff and her wrists, ankles, and knees were swollen. At first, this stiffness was worse in the morning and wore off during the day. However, it suddenly became much worse so that even at the end of the day she was dragging herself around. We tried chiropractic treatments, but although she felt better immediately after the treatment, the stiffness continued to get worse.

"We took her then to an MD. He took extensive blood and urine tests. He had her try taking large amounts of aspirin but this made her`dizzy. After about a week of tests, the doctor called my husband and me in for a conference. He said Judi's ailment had been diagnosed as lupus erythematosus, a rare disease that affects the connective tissue. He said the only treatment that had been found for it was cortisone and he started her on 60 mg. a day. The stiffness was gone almost immediately. (She was now starting her freshman year in high school.) She would come home from school exhausted. We realized that this was due in part to the fact that she had been inactive for so long but something else was bothering her. The doctor checked her blood and urine each week for a while, then every three weeks. He gradually lowered the amounts of cortisone. However, she continued to feel tired all the time and had constant headaches. Her face became puffy and she retained a lot of water. She gained twelve pounds and could not get into most of her clothes. The cortisone treatments were started in September. By April the amount had been cut down to 5 mg. a day and we were looking forward to going off it entirely. Then, the symptoms started coming back; her joints began to get stiff again.

"It was just at this time that a friend happened to mention Dr. Nittler who treated patients through diet. We decided to try this rather than continue with the cortisone. Again there were many tests. Dr. Nittler found that Judi had hypoglycemia which results from the malfunction of the adrenal gland. The outward effect of this was the lupus erythematosus. The cortisone treated only the outer effects; he preferred to treat the source of the problem, and get the adrenal gland functioning properly again. He began giving her nutritional injections every week which gave the adrenal glands a rest. He took all carbohydrates and sugar out of her diet. She began to hold her own but was not improving too rapidly. So he put her on a completely raw food diet including a quart of carrot juice a day. She was also taking about seventy food supplements and vitamin pills a day. She began a gradual but sure and steady improvement. She is now beginning her sophomore year of high school. She can even swing a tennis racket without it hurting her wrist. She is now a normal, vibrant teenage girl enjoying life in high school."

CHAPTER VIII

DO-IT-YOURSELF NUTRITION

THIS CHAPTER is dedicated to timely and practical nutritional tips. When used with common sense these tips can be used as home remedies with little fear of complications. They are not a substitute for a nutritionally trained doctor, but are better than doing nothing at all or using questionable drugs.

This information is supplied for those of you who are forced to do things on your own. It can be very gratifying, though again, I urge you to use common sense.

Here are some helpful hints on treating common ailments at home.

Vitamin E and Your Heart

Vitamin E is good for heart conditions. It has three major functions: it increases blood flow volume and oxygen utilization in the local heart tissues and improves circulation throughout the body. People who complain of cold feet are often helped by vitamin E. It may also improve a poor memory. Because of the increased blood flow, the arterioles become relaxed or dilated and allow more blood to flow per minute to the brain, the heart muscle, as well as to other areas of the body. This function of blood flow plus increase of oxygen utilization automatically lowers the work load of the heart and respiratory systems.

All people have special needs for vitamin E which

must be determined by individual experimentation. I use three or four different brands and types of vitamin E. (See the end of this section for specific recommendations.) All are mixed tocopherols, or factors found in vitamin E, which are better in effect than larger amounts of one factor alone. The strongest factor is d-alpha tocopherol.

It is utterly stupid not to use vitamin E. No one knows in advance how much is best for you. You will have to experiment, week by week, beginning with a 100 I.U. (international unit) capsule, and working up, week by week, until you find the results desired. These results should include diminished symptoms, such as shortness of breath. Three hundred I.U. daily is a low average dose to take. Many people take 600 I.U. daily with excellent results and, in some cases, go as high or higher than 1,600 I.U. daily, although these high dosages are usually prescribed by vitamin E informed doctors who watch the patient carefully and set the dose accordingly. I personally take between 2,000 and 3,000 I.U. of mixed tocopherols per day.

There are three cautions to observe in taking vitamin E. One, if you have high blood pressure, it is necessary to start with a low dose and increase the amount week by week very cautiously. Your blood pressure may rise if high dosages are begun suddenly. The use of inorganic iron or female hormones cancels out vitamin E. The solution to this problem is to take vitamin E eight to twelve hours before or after the hormones and/or inorganic iron, if your doctor has prescribed them. You could take your vitamin E in the morning and the other medication at night, or vice versa.

It is also interesting, according to Wilfrid E. Shute, M.D. and Harold Taub in their book *Vitamin E for*

Ailing and Healthy Hearts* that vitamin E disappears from the blood stream entirely if it is discontinued for three days. Dr. Shute, with his brother, Evan Shute, M.D., both of Canada, have rehabilitated many thousands of damaged hearts over the years by the use of adequate amounts of vitamin E. The book by Dr. Wilfrid Shute with Harold Taub will give you more information on how this is done. The types of vitamin E I prescribe include:

Eeee Plus by Sunshine Valley
Super Eeee Plus by Sunshine Valley
Cataplex E by Vitamin Products Co.
(a subsidiary of Standard Process Labs)
Cataplex E-2 by Vitamin Products Co.
Denamone by Viobin

Constipation

Constipation is a great problem for many. I consider the best remedy an occasional, if necessary only, plain tap-water enema. An enema removes the debris without irritating the bowel. Continued enemas tend to be habit forming. However, an enema containing two tablespoonfuls each of lemon juice and honey per quart is detoxifying and stimulating.

It is always better to avoid constipation in the first place. A diet consistently high in raw foods is usually adequate for stimulating the bowels. Flax seed meal is excellent. Two tablespoonfuls of flax seed meal mixed in your cereal or juice each morning should do the job. Another temporary, simple means of stimulating the bowel without bad effects or irritation is to drink a quart of warm salt water before breakfast. Prepare the salt water by putting two teaspoonfuls of solar dried sea or earth salt into

*Pyramid Publications, New York, N.Y., 1970.

the quart bottle before adding the hot water to it.

If a laxative must be relied upon, the best one to take is castor oil, but only *through the skin and not by mouth.* Just use the oil as a body rub, especially over the abdomen. Use about two or three tablespoonfuls of castor oil, rubbing it in thoroughly. The results should be forthcoming the following morning. You might need a larger dosage. Trial will tell you what you need. A hot pad on the tummy after the massage helps.

Another simple herbal remedy which you can make for yourself is as follows:

First mix, then grind or pulverize in a blender:

3/4 oz. powdered senna leaves	3/4 oz. olive oil
	1/4 oz. glycerin
1/4 oz. powdered slippery elm bark	
1/2 oz. powdered charcoal	

(These products may be obtained in most drugstores.) Form into about 10 walnut-size balls. Grind:

3/4 lb. black mission figs (not treated with
    sulfur)
3/8 lb. raisins

(May be obtained from health food stores.) Mix thoroughly and roll the balls in the fig-raisin mixture to coat them.

Eat one ball every day, preferably before breakfast, until they work. Half or quarter portions may be used as indicated.

Diarrhea

As you know, diarrhea is a condition where there are frequent watery bowel movements. The cause varies. It can be due to anything from food poisoning to infections or, occasionally, something more serious. However, diarrhea is potentially very serious because of acute and/or chronic loss of fluids, beneficial intestinal flora, B vitamins, minerals and electrolytes from the intestines.

The first thing to do is to stop eating, even to the point of taking no water until the diarrhea stops. If it does not stop quickly, you can replace some of the minerals by rubbing into the skin a solution of 2 teaspoonfuls of apple cider vinegar and 1 teaspoonful of solar dried earth or sea salt combined in one glassful of water. In emergencies, where high fever exists, this skin feeding can be a continuous procedure. Otherwise, four times daily will suffice.

Another remedy is to use simmered skim milk (skim milk just brought to a boil); take one glassful four times daily. Eat it like soup; use a spoon so that you drink it slowly.

Barley water can be used as an alternative: boil 5 cupfuls of water then add 1 cupful of barley grains. Simmer twenty minutes. Strain off fluid and drink. Repeat this four times daily.

Powdered carob mixed in water (available at health stores), 1-2 teaspoonfuls per glass, will usually stop diarrhea in short order. Dosage may be repeated as often as necessary.

Diarrhea is the result of a bowel irritation that the body is trying to eliminate. Sometimes, if all else fails, hydrochloric acid will do the job.

A supplement of great value is *Cholacol II* by Standard Process Laboratories. It contains bile salts and clay. Take four of these tablets after each water bowel movement until relieved.

Kaopectate ® by Upjohn Company, from the drugstore, is another clay remedy. Take as directed.

All these remedies are far better for you than drugs.

Gallbladder Colic

Acute gallbladder colic is extremely painful. It usually means you are trying to pass a gallstone. It responds poorly, if at all, to such remedies as aspirin, phenacetin and even codeine or morphine. Hotpads, massage and other adjuncts are of little avail.

However, there is a simple, temporary remedy; the coffee enema. Percolate a strong cupful of coffee. Important: neither instant nor decaffeinated coffee is acceptable. It must be brewed natural coffee. Dilute this strong cupful of coffee to 1 pint with water (do not add sugar and cream). Use this as a retention enema, i.e., hold in rectum as long as possible.

The coffee enema causes a relaxation in the liver-gallbladder region which gives rapid relief of pain. If you are lucky, you could even pass a gallstone or two. Maybe more. If you are not lucky, the pain returns and you must repeat the process until help can arrive for more definitive care. In either event, you have jeopardized nothing.

This is the one and only time I recommend coffee. As a drink, it is a no-no for hypoglycemics, which applies to most people.

Another remedy is the use of epsom salts: 1/2 tsp. in water at bedtime or *Fleet's PhosphoSoda* ®, at drugstores, 1/4 tsp. in water at bedtime. Either can do wonders in stimulating the flow of bile from the liver and gallbladder. *Betaris* by Standard Process Laboratories, a tablet made from powdered beet top juice, causes the density or S.A.E. of the bile to be reduced, thus making it more flowable. Increased flowability of bile in sluggish gallbladders can be very beneficial. Sometimes the formation of the gallstones can even be reversed.

Heartburn and Ulcers

Heartburn is a very common ailment. Many people eat too much of the wrong foods and suffer the consequences. It is a burning sensation in the pit of the stomach, in the inverted V between the ribs in front. It comes, usually, a short time after meals.

Antacids work on a temporary basis, only until the next time. In the meanwhile, the antacids grossly upset the normal acid-alkaline balance in the whole system, not only the stomach. Of course, the acidity of the stomach is immediately neutralized or even made alkaline by ingestion of antacids. This means that your stomach protein digestion processes immediately stop. Acidity in the lower intestines is necessary for proper absorption but is disturbed by antacid therapy. Even the normal pH of the blood is adversely affected by the hyperalkaline intestinal contents which are being absorbed.

So you see, taking antacids is not without eventual harmful consequences.

In reality, most, but not all, cases of heartburn are due not to too much acid, as TV commercials would have you believe, but to *lack* of stomach acid. The symptoms of too much and too little acid are identical. There is a very simple test: drink a solution of apple cider or wine vinegar (2 tsp. in 1 glassful of water) when you have heartburn. If you get almost immediate relief, your need is for more acid and not for antacids. If the vinegar intake aggravates the heartburn, your need is for the antacid, which can then be taken with no added risk to your stomach.

Oddly enough, where an ulcer or pre-ulcer state exists, initially the basic need may have been for more acid. Lack of it may have caused the glands in the stomach wall to overwork and eventually resulted in a breakdown of the stomach lining. When this has happened, any acid then becomes too much and antacids are needed. This is true even though eventual cure depends upon reestablishment of proper acid function in the stomach.

The secret of successful therapy is to be able to get more acid into the system without causing an aggravation of the local stomach symptoms. This demands individualized therapy. A nutritious, easily digestible, high protein diet is basic. The diet will provide the body with the essential building blocks which are necessary for repair. The protein must be in a form for easy digestion. Protein powders derived from milk are a great help here. Frequent smaller feedings lower the chance of overproduction of acid at any one time. Vitamin C taken with food, not on an empty stomach, to aid healing is a must. Other nutrients are added slowly to the program as the stomach begins to heal. Then, with the course set and no symptoms present, just keep going to allow two to four weeks for adequate healing. Slow and easy is the order of the day. Do not rush stomach healing therapy.

A capsule of great value is *Comfrey-Pepsin* by Standard Process Laboratories. This substance has a wonderful healing effect on the mucous membranes of the intestinal tract. The sticky comfrey holds the pepsin against the mucus stomach lining to aid healing. One capsule, as often as needed, even hourly, can perform miracles in a short time when combined with the proper diet.

Hemorrhoids — Intestinal Parasites

Hemorrhoids can be very painful and unpleasant. The usual medical approach to such a problem is surgery. This approach is based on the assumption that what is no longer there cannot bother you. Such a philosophy absolutely ignores the cause; it concerns only the symptoms.

However, there is a simpler, more natural approach. One must consider a twofold cause: (1) weakness of local venous structure, and (2) liver problems.

The use of *Collinsonia* root powder capsules (by Standard Process Laboratories) can be very helpful. The dosage can vary but is quite safe, in fact, virtually without side effects. If you really have a problem, take one capsule hourly. Less severe cases can use one or two capsules three times daily. Benefit should be apparent in a day or less, though cure may not result for a few weeks. Cure is directly related to improved liver function. Continue a maintenance dose for a couple of months for insurance. You should be able to discontinue other medication without recurrence of the problem.

The insertion of a peeled garlic bud or a suppository made of raw potato also may bring relief.

Rectal itching may be an early warning of the development of hemorrhoids. It can also be a symptom of too little hydrochloric acid or the presence of intestinal parasites. An itch is a warning that something is not right. It is early evidence of localized malnutrition. It is easy to use a capsule made from figs containing enzymes (*Zymex II* by Standard Process Laboratories) which digest the worms. One or two capsules three times daily for a two- to three-month period should do the job. If results are more urgent, one could take one capsule on an hourly basis for twenty-four hours while fasting. Start the day with a colonic or an enema. Nothing but salty water, made by adding 1 teaspoonful of solar dried sea or earth salt to 1 quart of water, is allowed during the whole day. A three-a-day dosage for a month should easily finish off the parasites.

If the itch is of unknown origin, you could try the use of *Noxzema* ® by Noxzema Chemicals Company, at drugstores, applying the cream with a tissue to the anal area. The tissue may be gently tucked into place for the night. Do this for a few nights and you will find great relief.

Spray Residue

Most of us have difficulty obtaining real organic, unsprayed produce. The sprays appear on the surface of the produce but are also built into the food through the root system of the plants. There is no way to remove the built-in contaminants. There are measures which can remove the surface spray from all vegetables and fruits grown above ground. These are the foods which have been exposed directly to planes and other forms of crop dusting and spraying.

To remove surface accumulation, soak the produce (separate the leaves or stalks of lettuce, celery, cabbage and artichokes to reach the embedded residue) in a dishpan in which 2-1/2 teaspoons of 10 percent dilute hydrochloric acid (available at drugstores) have been added to 1 quart of water; or 2 tablespoons of apple cider vinegar to the entire dishpanful of water. Soak the produce for about twenty minutes and then rinse.

A way to avoid sprayed food is to use sprouted seeds. Choose wheat, radish, mung beans, alfalfa or any others you wish and sprout them yourself. It is easy and the sprouts are extremely rich in vitamins and minerals as well as being raw, which is a benefit to health. Soak the seeds overnight. In the morning, pour off the water and place the seeds between several layers of white paper towels placed in a colander. Soak the towels and seeds by holding the colander under the running faucet. After draining, put away on the corner of your kitchen counter. In the morning, reirrigate. In a few days you will have a crop of sprouts to add to salads, sandwiches, or dropped into soups or omelets *after* these dishes have been cooked so the sprouts will not be cooked and many of their nutrients will not be destroyed. Sprouts can be kept in a plastic bag in the refrigerator for several days.

Do not buy seeds which have been chemically coated from feed stores. Purchase the plain, natural seeds at health stores.

Toothbrushing

The best way to brush your teeth is to massage the gums thoroughly with a soft natural bristle toothbrush. Do not merely wave the toothbrush over the teeth. This waving maneuver does not massage the gums. Use dental floss to release debris from between the teeth. A good gum scrubbing, then, is all that is needed. It is not even necessary to use a dentifrice. Most dentifrices contain harmful chemicals. These chemicals not only can weaken and scratch the enamel but also destroy the normal bacterial flora in the mouth which, in turn, interferes with the normal flora throughout the whole intestinal tract. A disturbed intestinal flora spells nothing but trouble. A soft bristled toothbrush with nothing on it is the best and all anyone needs along with the dental floss. If you feel you *must* use some sort of cleansing material, you can try a little solar dried sea or earth salt. This provides taste as well as providing the trace minerals found in nature. I do not recommend soda for this purpose since it is chemically lopsided in favor of sodium, which is excessively alkaline. There are some good dentifrices found in health food stores made from various natural substances. One is a papaya powder which is very good. Another is Moor's from Germany. It contains trace minerals.

Apple Cider Vinegar

Most of us have heard of apple cider vinegar as a wonderful folk medicine remedy. So it is, in many instances.

In my experience, I have found that an apple cider vinegar rub (use it straight just as you would rubbing alcohol) can do wonders for patients with a fever. Children respond exceptionally well. The rule of thumb is to rub them down with apple cider vinegar as often as needed to bring the fever down to normal. It may mean continuous rubbing, or 15-to-30-minute, or longer, intervals. Whatever is needed is the proper dosage. It may take up to a few hours to effect results but it is worth the effort. You will easily recognize the results because the patient goes through a sort of crisis. He then settles down comfortably. Even if it does not entirely solve the problem and further care is needed, you have not lost anything in trying and could have gained much. Apple cider vinegar will not interfere with any other type of therapy. It actually feeds the body through the skin: mainly, potassium and acid. Both of these substances are especially needed during acute illness.

Hot vs. Cold Treatment

When confronted with the decision as to whether to use hot or cold compresses on the body, you should first understand a little basic physiology. When an infection is in the system it can represent one of three stages of inner-body war: a beginning; in full progress; or in the process of being defeated.

Application of heat speeds up the whole activity, both bacterial and bodily, while ice slows them down. If the infection is ahead in the war, heat will make your problem worse. If the body defense system is ahead, the infection will subside. Cold slows the activity, thus buying time while the body develops more resistance. One must use common sense. You might even use alternate ten-minute compresses of hot, then ice, when the circumstances are right.

When in doubt, use ice. You cannot get into trouble this way.

The best and most ancient method of inducing healing of an infected wound on the fingers or hands is to suck on it. While gently sucking, the tongue can play with the lesion. A few short sessions of mouth therapy usually effects a rapid cure. Animals do this instinctively.

Prostate Congestion

Prostate congestion is a common complaint of the aging male. He begins to note that it is difficult for him to empty his bladder. He notes that the morning stream is less forceful; it takes longer for the bladder to empty; and it empties less well. There may be night-time urination. Night leg nervousness is an associated complaint. These are a few of the signs and symptoms.

There is an exercise which can be used as you lie on the bed before retiring which can help to relieve the condition. To do this correctly, lie flat on your back, pull the knees up as far as possible, then put the soles of the feet together. Holding this sole-to-sole position as forcefully as possible, gradually extend the legs. Naturally, at some point the soles no longer touch, but a little practice will enhance your ability. Each repetition of this exercise gives the

prostate a good squeeze. It is a do-it-yourself prostatic massage. Repeat the exercise one hundred times
a day or whatever you can manage for a start.

Two types of nutritional tablets have proven to be
of great value to countless patients. They are *Prostate Cytotrophin* by Standard Process Laboratories
and *Cataplex F* by Vitamin Products Company (a subsidiary of Standard Process Lab), both to be taken
three times daily.

It is fairly well known that eating squash seeds
also aids the normal function of the prostate gland.

Intercostal Neuralgia

Intercostal neuralgia is a condition where the
nerve or nerves between certain ribs are sending
pain sensations into the brain. It can feel as if your
chest is collapsing and it may be mistaken for a heart
attack, angina pectoris, coronary occlusion or even
acute gallbladder colic. It often happens when a
person is bending over. Since it frequently involves
the left side of the chest, the mistaken heart diagnosis can result. The simplest means of deciding the
difference is to determine if the skin and/or rib-cage
tissues are painful. Sometimes, even gentle probing
of the area with the finger elicits excruciating pain.
At other times, there are trigger areas of pain between ribs. Usually one intercostal nerve is involved.
In this case, the examiner can find a very tender trigger area just to one side of the sternum or breast
bone. As the interspace is followed around with the
finger, another trigger area can be found under the
arm and a third one just to the side of the spine, all
in the same interspace. The search will locate the
nerve involved.

Emergency treatment can be very simple. Ethyl
chloride may be used to freeze a strip of skin just to

the side of the spine starting about four inches above the located trigger point. Hold the bottle of ethyl chloride about three feet away and spray the spot until the skin spot freezes. Then extend the frozen spot downwards to make it a frozen strip about eight inches long. This frozen strip of skin breaks the reflex cycle between the pain area and the central nervous system. One treatment may tell if this is working for you. At any rate, it does buy time in which to get definitive nutritional therapy underway. Unfortunately, this freezing technique can sometimes cause a slight permanent pigmented line where the skin has been frostbitten.

In an emergency situation, when you cannot get ethyl chloride, ice can be of value when it is rubbed into the strictly defined area alongside the spine. Keep the ice localized in the predetermined area and do not let it wander. Diffuse chilling could nullify the reflex-breaking power of the cold.

Sometimes large doses of calcium lactate can alleviate this type of pain. Continued calcium in the diet tends to disperse the pain.

Colds and Flu

What to do for the flu? Since we are all subject to epidemics of the flu, we should have a preestablished plan of action.

The use of lecithin is fantastic. Take 1 tablespoon of liquid lecithin, or sixty 200-mg. perles, or ten 1,200-mg. capsules four times daily for six doses for quick relief of early virus infections. This remedy alone cures many cases of flu. Liquid lecithin or perles are available at health stores. Warning: lecithin is a phospholipid, high in phosphorus and can cause acute calcium shortage if this high dosage is continued. If you need more than one series of lecithin, be sure to compensate with large doses of nonphosphorus calcium, such as calcium lactate.

This lecithin routine can be used for any virus infection, such as measles, shingles, chicken pox.

If the lecithin fails, which happens sometimes, the following program may be followed:

1. Vitamin C (even synthetic ascorbic acid will do), 1,000 mg.

2. Cataplex A by Vitamin Products Company

3. Calcium lactate by Standard Process Laboratories; 41 mg. tablet

4. Kelp or sponge tablet (*Iodomere* by Standard Process Laboratories)

Take one of each of these tablets on an hourly basis while awake. Drink copious amounts of spring water and thin juices, but no solid food. Take an enema using 2 tablespoonfuls each of lemon juice and honey. Have an apple cider vinegar body rub hourly. This combination should cure your cold in short order. Continue the regimen for several days to insure a cure. Warning: iodine in kelp or sponge will cause nervousness when overdosed. Unfortunately, the therapeutic dose for flu becomes an overdose as soon as you feel better. Be alert to the cut-off point. At worst, you might not sleep well for a night.

For colds 1,000 mg. of ascorbic acid plus one calcium lactate tablet every hour will *prevent*, not cure, a cold if taken immediately on the first symptoms of scratchy throat, sneezing, etc.

One thing of great importance which most of us neglect is to treat a cold with bed rest. Take time off to allow your body to heal.

Cough

A nagging cough is very annoying not only to the one who coughs but also to the listeners. Cough syrups, found in the drugstores, are a sugar-based medication, as indicated by the name "syrup." They are saturated with sugar in order to disguise the taste of the medication. I sometimes wonder if it isn't just the sugar that relieves the cough.

However, those of us who wish to avoid refined sugar and drugs can readily do so. A simple formula to use is a mixture of 1/2 cupful of fresh lemon juice and 1/2 cupful honey. A third equal portion of glycerine *for internal use only* may be used if desired. Mix these thoroughly, then take about 3 teaspoonfuls every ten minutes until the cough subsides. Depending upon the individual problem, the cough will be relieved for an hour or more. Repeat the routine as needed. Naturally, it does not work as efficiently for as long a time as the drug types, but remember, it is not a drug. We can well afford this sort of inconvenience in order to avoid drugs.

To ease nasal congestion, use a vaporizer such as those used for children, adding one teaspoonful of tincture of benzoin compound per pint of water. The vaporizer can be used off and on for twenty minutes four times daily or more. It can even be used all night. The humidity in the atmosphere containing tincture of benzoin compound tends to prevent the nasal secretions from getting dried out, sticky and difficult to remove. It is this sticky, glue-type mucus that frequently causes the nagging cough, which is an inefficient attempt to expectorate a small amount of sticky mucus. A vaporizer treatment guards against this.

Your vaporizing apparatus can be easily cleaned by using distilled vinegar as a solvent after using the tincture of benzoin compound.

Athlete's Foot

Athlete's foot is a type of fungus infection commonly affecting the toes and feet. It usually defies treatment. It is always existent in public showers.

However, the use of Trapper's Ointment* may produce gratifying results. This is an herbal ointment which can be applied locally in a small to moderate amount and then massaged into the skin thoroughly covering the whole foot or area involved.

I have known very severe long-standing cases to respond dramatically after one application. Of course, this is not always 100 percent effective, but it usually is quite efficient.

Boils or Other Acute Infections

It is true that the boils or other types of acute skin conditions are the result of the body trying to get rid of accumulated poisons. The drainage should not be stopped but should be enhanced and the cause eliminated. This is one of the drawbacks of antibiotic therapy: antibiotics stop the infections locally, i.e. the local drainage, but the basic cause of the infection has not been solved; the local tissue malnutrition has not been corrected. A simple compress can be of great value in getting rid of boils. A compress made from papaya is excellent. In fact, a compress made from figs, raw grated potatoes, pineapple, melons, bread, onions or garlic all have value. Just mash some of the material onto a gauze pad and apply this to the lesion overnight. If you think you might be allergic to any of these, check your skin with small band-aid size compresses before using large compresses. I have seen a deep nasty boil on a cheek drain through the skin in one night with the use of the papaya compress: the exudate was on the pad, there was no exudate left in the boil and

*Available through Baker's International Distributors, P.O. Box 736, Boise, Idaho 83701.

there was no evidence as to how it passed through the skin. Amazing, you say. I agree. But try it and see.

Burns

The first thing to do when there is a skin burn is to apply ice. Cover the whole area as quickly and as thoroughly as possible. I remember a small child who had pulled the coffee pot over onto herself. I gave orders to apply ice as quickly as possible. This was done but not thoroughly enough. Later when the damage could be surveyed, one could see islands of healthy tissue in the middle of the burn just the shape of the ice cubes where they had been applied.

The next first-aid remedy is to sponge the area with salt water. Do this by mixing 2 teaspoonfuls of solar dried sea or earth salt in a quart of water and apply this to the wound with a large cotton wad. Keep the area moist with the salt solution.

One doctor tells of a case where there was approximately 80 percent of the body covered with first and second degree burns. Ordinarily this means there is no hope for the patient. The doctor used large doses of vitamin C orally and intravenously, even 30- 40,000 mg. daily, as well as repeated spraying of the burned area with a 3 percent solution of ascorbic acid. This man recovered with only a small scarred area in one armpit where it had been necessary to leave a gauze pad as a dressing. Otherwise, the wounds were left wide open and sprayed frequently. There was practically no residual scar.

Keep an *Aloe vera* plant in your garden or on your kitchen windowsill. Cut off an inch, squeeze out or rub the plant's jelly onto the burn. Presto! The pain goes and leaves no scars. Puncturing a vitamin E capsule and repeatedly applying it to old burn scars eventually minimizes them. Taking vitamin E internally may also dramatically speed healing. Vitamin F ointment also tends to minimize old scars.

Poison Oak, Ivy

Poison oak or ivy produce a very uncomfortable allergic reaction. It is a self-limiting disease because it will not last very long. There is a very simple remedy which can lighten your burden greatly. Simply take large doses of vitamin C. I would suggest a dosage like 2,000 or 3,000 mg. hourly until relief is in sight. Then the interval can be prolonged or the amount reduced according to the need. Using sea water and sun to dry out the lesions is another great aid in getting relief. Go ocean swimming, if possible, and bask in the sun for a short while. If these are not possible, you can use some apple cider vinegar as a body rub over the areas involved. As the rash dries, the vinegar can be rubbed in more and more vigorously. This shortens the total drying period.

Two natural remedies which may be helpful are the plants *Dusty Miller* and *Aloe vera*. The *Dusty Miller* is to be crushed and macerated and made into a cold tea. The tea may be applied directly to the lesion. With the *Aloe vera*, the leaf is opened to expose the watery gel interior. The watery gel is applied directly to the poison oak for very soothing relief; or tea made by boiling bay (laurel) leaves in water can be applied to the poison oak or ivy rash for its anti-itch and drying effect.

Finally, the use of the homeopathic remedy, *Rhus Tox*, will be of value in the acute phase as well as preventing it by taking *before* the poison oak-ivy season, thus providing an immunity program.

Warts

Castor oil is derived from the bean of the castor plant. This plant is called, colloquially, the Palm of

Christ because of the shape of the leaf and because of the benefits obtained from it.

Many different types of skin lesions respond to application of castor oil. Skin tabs, commonly known as meat balls, may melt away with persistent application of the castor oil. So will seed warts. Even the regular warts will decrease in size and sometimes completely disappear. Large lesions like senile and seborrheic keratoses improve under this treatment. In fact, I would try using castor oil on any skin lesion for a reasonable period before subjecting to surgical treatment. One or two applications per day are sufficient for most purposes. It may even help remove brown spots. Castor oil does not work on these skin conditions overnight. One patient used it on a large, unsightly face wart, rubbing it in every night. One year later, the wart was gone.

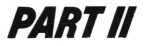

PART II

INTRODUCTION TO PART II

PART II is really intended for physicians. It contains technical information which doctors understand. If you are interested in how hypoglycemia can be detected and controlled, and how other diseases can be arrested or reversed by nutritional therapy, by all means read it. You will certainly enjoy the case histories presented in Chapter X.

I suggest that you take this book to your doctor and ask him to read it *all*, not just Part II. My own patients were responsible for getting me started in metabolic nutrition, and I hope your doctor will be open-minded enough to begin the use of nutritional therapy in his practice, too. If you wish to skip the technical information in Part II, for doctors, I will not blame you. But I will be disappointed if you do not take the book to your doctor so that he can learn to help you and others by this new method. Do not leave it with him indefinitely. Set a deadline, a week or two. Tell him at which time you will pick it up. Otherwise, he may never read it! He is a busy person, and may not otherwise allow himself time.

Do not blame your doctor too much for not knowing about hypoglycemia, or nutritional therapy for treating other ailments. It probably was not taught him when he was in medical school. Therefore, as a few other physicians and I have done, he may have to learn how to use this new method on his own. You can help by introducing it to him. If he is not interested *after* a fair perusal of the book (don't merely ask him if he will read it, since he will say no on first impulse), take it to another doctor until you find one who does show positive interest after he has read it.

Treating patients nutritionally is not the only problem. The physician, himself, should remain in good health so that he can care for those who need his help. He is a human being, too, with a body subject to the same ills and even greater stresses, often, than his patients. He needs to keep well. Nutritional therapy can be invaluable to him.

So we need a new breed of doctor in these times of deteriorating national health. If you, the patient, can encourage him, perhaps this dream can come true. I pray that it will.

CHAPTER IX

HOW TO LEARN NUTRITIONAL KNOW-HOW

As I HAVE mentioned previously, there is no place to go for formal nutritional education. No approved medical institution looks favorably upon this subject. The usual medical curriculum includes some 4,000 total hours of medical education and only from zero to five credit hours of so-called nutrition, which is in reality dietetics, an entirely different subject. What is taught mainly includes such things as low sodium diets for hypertension, bland diets for ulcers, low cholesterol diets for arterial and heart problems and calorie counting for obesity. All are sadly out of date by newer nutritional standards, and what's more, the public knows it! They are fed up with palliative measures and are losing confidence in the average medical practitioner and the drugs he uses to cover up symptoms. They are watching others, laymen and a *few* doctors, who are reversing illness. They (the public) are beginning to do the same things themselves through the newer concept of nutrition which teaches that the body is only as strong as what is put into it. Like a building, or a bridge, the body will endure stress and strain only if it is made of the best materials, of which the baby was created in the first place. These materials must be kept in constant supply in order to maintain good health. The public is reading, learning and using this approach with great success. There is no need for physicians to lose face during this revolution, which, believe me, is not temporary. My advice is, if you can't beat them, join them! Do as some doctors are already doing: educate yourself nutritionally. I will give you some tips on how to get started.

Many physicians recommend a good nutritious diet for their patients when they themselves have neither been trained nor even have the faintest idea what a good nutritious diet is! One young physician told me he believed that the body could get all the nutrients it needs from hot dogs, french fries and Cokes, so long as the person is kept free from hunger. Frankly, this man has a lot to learn. I could fill an entire page in this book with names of the chemicals and body disturbing elements found in these items alone which may be stomach fillers but not body builders. Colorings, dyes, chemicals galore replace any nutrients which once may have existed in these foods but now add up only to a bunch of chemicals. Many of these very chemicals have been found to be cancer-causing in experimental situations.

I realize that the average doctor is beset by suspicions about nutrition. He has been warned it is quackery or faddism. A small percentage of it may be, but there is also a mass of growing research from laboratories the world over which is not quackery. Why do people fall for it indiscriminately? Because, they have no doctor to guide them. They have to learn the hard way for themselves. Even at that, it may be safer for the patient in the long run than the doctor's use of experimental drugs. All too often these experimental drugs become demoted, one by one, because of their dangerous side effects. Let's face it, brainwashing takes place in the drug field as in any other. At least the nutritional fads won't kill people. People are clamoring for doctors who can separate the nutritional truths from the untruths so they won't have to experiment on themselves. At present, they are now learning by trial and error, by the hundreds of thousands. This army is increasing daily!

True science must develop demonstrable facts, not just opinions based on medical consensus. Testing can be tricky. To begin with, many tests are performed in subsidized laboratories which are trying to slant the results for ulterior reasons. Nutritional testing is especially difficult because there are so many variables. For instance, a test of a nutritional substance may fail because too small a dosage was used for too short a time. The false or incomplete verdict is then announced that the product is of no value. This has happened in the case of vitamins E and C. Both of these vitamins were rejected by the medical profession, but not the public, who used them with great success. In spite of attempts to slander or eliminate them, these vitamins have now become, when properly used, both accepted and successful. True science must be entirely objective and without bias.

The public is now ahead of the doctors and is taking the bit in its teeth. The once respected, almost worshiped, medical profession is rapidly losing its public image. I repeat, the solution is: if you can't beat the opposition, in this case the unsatisfied public, join it! A joiner can become a leader. I realize that the average doctor is wary. He has spent years of his life learning the allopathic approach. He feels secure in his field. Unfortunately allopathy is neither meeting the needs of today nor the demands of an ever-increasing intelligent public. You would be amazed how much more the layman knows about this subject than the doctor. Even the press has discovered how important, as well as how popular, the subject of nutrition is to the general public, and is reporting laboratory findings as priority news. These reports are seized upon by a hungry public whose health is failing under the care of the busy, nutritionally unprepared and bewildered physician.

The only way I know to meet this challenge and survive professionally is to allow some time in your reading of medical literature for reading and studying nutritional literature. Read, study, learn. Attend any "health" conventions in your vicinity. Sure, you will find some crackpots, but you will also find other lecturers who have discovered nutritional truths which do work. You may shudder at the lack of education, as you know it, of some of these people who may not know the meaning of the word "documentation," and couldn't care less. They may just have rediscovered a natural remedy upon which some of our early pharmacology was based but is now banned in favor of more expensive drugs. Watch the people in the audience. Hear their testimonies. Pay attention to any of the outstanding well-educated experts in the field of nutrition who are devoting their lives to nutritional research and using it clinically with tremendous success. There may be only one or a few in this category at a convention because they are rare, overworked and hard to come by for public lecturing. They may have an M.A., a Ph.D., a D.D.S. or an M.D., so don't underrate their intelligence. They are merely educated in a field in which you are not but should be. The public is following them like Pied Pipers because they not only promise better health but they deliver it! Nutritional reporters often make reports on scientific studies and practical concepts many years before the ideas are actually accepted by contemporary medicine. Acceptance usually comes only after a battle with the status quo. In getting your postgraduate education, don't be afraid to listen to a lecture or read a book by a "crackpot." You might learn something, even only one point of importance. I have been called both "crackpot" and "beloved physician."

After you read and listen, and I implore you to do both with an open mind, then begin to experiment. A little now and a little later is enough at first. Try nutrition on yourself, as I did. You can expect some surprises. As you gain confidence, add more nutritional tools to your trade. If you are a specialist, try it in your specialty. I know of several physicians who have been amazed with the increased success of the nutritional vs. the drug approach in their particular fields. Don't give up if you have a failure. Try to learn why it did not work and keep trying. Believe me, you have no need to fear that your practice will fall off. The nutritional M.D.'s I know are so swamped with delighted patients that they are establishing more confidence than ever. The word-of-mouth publicity is bringing a never-ending line up to their doors.

Where can you find such information? I list the sources I know of at the end of this chapter.

As you add to your nutritional knowledge, you will wonder what products are the best to use. I have tried many. I have definitely rejected the synthetics, except in a few situations for temporary control only. I have found that whole, truly natural supplements, not just those products which pretend to be natural, bring the best results in the long run. I have finally settled down to a few sources, though I am not absolutely rigid about clinging to these alone. New and good products, as well as questionable ones, are coming out all the time. I try to keep alert for the good ones. If they measure up, I add them to my armamentarium.

The ones which have better stood the test of time for me are those made by Standard Process Labs., with a subsidiary, Vitamin Products Co., located in Milwaukee, Wisconsin 53201. They were formulated by the late Dr. Royal Lee, D.D.S., who was an outstanding leader in the nutritional movement. One M.D., highly knowledgeable in the nutritional field himself, states that he considered Dr. Lee, whom he knew personally, the best-informed person on nutrition in America, perhaps even the world. Dr. Lee originally became interested in nutrition as a preventive method for treatment of dental caries. During his career he researched the world's nutritional literature. He then began to try to find products with the qualifications necessary to match the scientific nutritional studies. He soon learned that there were no such products at that time which he considered reliable. So he proceeded to produce them himself. Many times there were no tools or machines to do the job so he invented them. For example, he invented a vacuum dehydrator which is still in operation. Ultimately, he founded a company, now Standard Process Labs. with its subsidiary, Vitamin Product Co. These companies still produce, according to his formulas, nutritional supplements of the highest standards. The products are among the finest supplements known and are usually available through doctors only. Because they are so trustworthy and helpful I use them very extensively in my practice. I keep them on hand in my office for convenience and dispense them to my patients as needed.

As you encounter various names of products in the case histories offered below for you to consider, they often, but not always, are from this source. There are other excellent products, including the chelated minerals, which come from other companies. Nothing should be excluded if it will do the job.

Before I list some suggested reading to help you in your postgraduate nutritional education, let us here and now dispel some myths. As you scan the names of the authors, you may react against some of them because you have been led to believe they are "quacks," "faddists" or "health nuts." I assure you they are not or I would not have listed their publications. I have urged patients in Part I to use a little common sense in handling their health problems naturally. I urge you, as a doctor, to use common sense in making judgments about something or someone about whom you have *heard* or read derogatory remarks. Let's face it, there is usually a reason for continuous attacks, often unwarranted, on new methods, procedures or remedies. This *is* the history of medicine! When you have been warned again and again that a person or a remedy is useless or dangerous, put on your own thinking cap. Why did the government insist for so long that insecticides were perfectly safe, when they are now forced to admit that they are killing off wild life, upsetting our ecology and are also poisonous, even carcinogenic, for people? Did it ever occur to you that the chemical insecticide industry may have been playing footsies with certain members of government agencies to prevent the publication of such information, which would be a large burden financially?

Why has the government insisted for so long that this country does not suffer from malnutrition, as preached by some governmental spokesmen, while others in the same bureau have conducted respected research with contrary conclusions? The government finally was forced to admit this discrepancy. Could it be that the food processors, who claim that our food is the best in the world and that natural foods, vitamins, minerals, etc. found in health foods are useless, are robbing the public of millions óf dollars for worthless foods? Could it be that these health stores, which more and more people are patronizing while searching for unsprayed foods or whole foods untampered by man, are a financial threat to the food processing industry?

Don't cringe at the thought of health food stores. True, they are not perfect and everything they carry is not a "health food." They were sold a bill of goods, for instance, on the cyclamates by the manufacturers who supplied other stores, too. These stores try to live up to their stated purpose. To my knowledge they are the only sources of natural grains, other organic foods and natural supplements. The personnel, it is true, are often not educated according to our standards. In their defense, however, they still may know more about the natural health field than doctors. They operate these stores, or did at least until recently, because they themselves have experienced improvement in health through nutritional methods. They are trying to spread the message to others. The propaganda that they are rolling in money is ridicuous. Except for the few large stores, most—and this also includes some mail-order businesses—are operating on a shoestring. The products they sell, particularly the fragile natural produce and grains, are hand-processed, making them more expensive than machinery and mass produced and man-tampered foods. In order to make a profit at all, they have to add a 30 percent buffer to cover overhead costs. Yet, in spite of competition from supermarket prices, they manage to stay alive because people are searching for quality.

It is true that a change is taking place. The revolution I spoke of earlier, in which the public is becoming fighting mad because they have been hoodwinked by pesticide-doused and chemically laden processed foods, is in full sway. They are taking matters into their own hands and surging into the health stores and organic food markets in self-defense. It is about time. Other retailers, who previously spurned such foods, now see that they are in the minority and have decided to get on the bandwagon to make a fast buck. Some are labeling foods "natural" which are not natural, and produce "organic" which is not organic. Real discrimination, label reading and protective standards are now necessary to offset this food prostitution.

Did you ever wonder why information about the healing effects of natural herbs were belittled? The true claims made for the use of these simple, harmless herbs, fresh from the garden or forest, are causing many herbs to be banned. Golden Seal is a recent example. Let us hope this ban is temporary. Did you know that those who have made claims have been put behind bars even though many drugs include derivatives from these same herbs? Did it ever occur to you that following the announcement by Linus Pauling, a scientist and Nobel Prize winner, concerning his findings with vitamin C for colds, the rash of counterclaims, name-calling, and pooh-poohs against vitamin C might have resulted because Mr. Pauling stated that cold drug-remedies were useless? Did it ever occur to you that the drug industry will stop at nothing to remove competition which threatens its financial structure? Now that the highly touted Pill is falling into disrespect, on which the drug companies made billions and fought tooth and nail any attempts to discredit it, they are announcing, almost daily, hopeful substitutions in an attempt to recover their high profit status.

We doctors live in glass houses. I am reminded

of the science editor of a highly respected literary publication who, on seeing several doctors' names used as endorsement for some new "wonder drug" in an ad in a professional magazine, became suspicious. He wrote to these physicians at the addresses given. The letters were returned with the notation "No such address." For physicians who need to have office addresses and phone numbers so that their patients can reach them, this was somewhat mysterious. The science editor then tried to reach these men by phone and telegram. Same answer. It turned out that *there were no such doctors!* Their endorsement had been faked merely to convince other doctors that they should buy and use these drugs on their patients.

I will no doubt be taken to task for telling you the truth and there will be attempts to discredit this book. However, I have already had it. One more blow will not stop me. Other forms of persecution, including unsavory articles in medical magazines and the loss of membership in the AMA have not stopped me. The public is now aware. They are beginning to catch on to what is happening and to fight our battles for us who dare to rebel against such domination.

Again, I assure you, that if you have been "brainwashed" that the following authors are quacks because they dare to tell the truth about the natural health movement, nutrition and what both can accomplish, brush away the cobwebs of prejudice and reevaluate your thinking. For example, Adelle Davis, a leader in this field, is NOT an uneducated quack. She studied at Purdue University, Columbia University, the University of California, and has a master's of science degree from the University of Southern California Medical School. She served as a dietitian at Bellevue Hospital in New York City, and as supervisor of health education in the public school system of Yonkers, New York. Her successful nutritional clinical practice, which she has now abandoned in favor of writing, was gratefully received by thousands.

Linda Clark, nutrition reporter, has attended three universities and has a master's degree. With a few added hours of study she could be eligible for a Ph.D. She has rejected this higher degree because the prerequisites do not offer the research in nutrition she trusts and respects. So she has obtained the information on her own, without benefit of the Ph.D. In her first book, *Stay Young Longer,** she researched information for its contents for ten years in New York City's Academy of Medicine Library. She documented every finding stated in the book. This documented research was either conducted by a scientist, a physician or a laboratory in good standing. As a result this book is used as a textbook in several schools and universities. She will no longer reveal their names, because when she has, pressure is brought to bear on the schools (by guess who?) and the books have to go! Many public libraries have been asked to have a book-burning party for both Adelle Davis' and Linda Clark's books (again, by guess who?).

You may have heard denunciation of Carlton Fredericks, Ph.D. His only crime was to announce nutritional truths for fifteen years on his radio program which originated in New York City and was dedicated to educating people about nutrition. He is an expert on the subject. He denounced on the air such worthless foods as white bread and white sugar. He was called a liar and a crackpot (by guess who?) as he impressed his avid listeners. Yet, when Roger J. Williams, Ph.D., professor of chemistry at Univer-

*Pyramid Publications, New York, N.Y. Paperback. 1968.

sity of Texas, found recently that rats fed an exclusive diet of white bread died in approximately forty-five days, Carlton Fredericks' detractors ran for cover. Meanwhile he had already been thrown off some fifty radio stations in this country (by guess who?) for telling the truth.

I hope, by this time, you get the idea. You will get it still better if you will read these books, which represent years of respected nutritional research. They have been ignored by organized medical circles because they are controversial. This need not be. Nutrition could be a tremendous breakthrough to success for all doctors and patients.

Herewith a list of some of the available periodicals which can be read to obtain nutritional knowledge.

1. *American Journal of Clinical Nutrition:* Scientific nutritional investigation. 9650 Rockville Pike, Bethesda, Maryland 20014.

2. *Science:* Scientific papers on nutrition on occasion. American Association for the Advancement of Science, 1515 Massachusetts Avenue, N.W., Washington, D.C. 20005.

3. *Nutrition Abstracts & Reviews:* Review of world's literature on nutrition. Commonwealth Bureau of Animal Nutrition, Bucksburn, Aberdeen, AB2 9SB, Scotland.

4. *Journal International Academy of Applied Nutrition:* Nutritional research publication. International College of Applied Nutrition, Box 286, La Habra, California 90631.

5. *Nutrition Today:* Practical application of nutrition in medicine. Enloe, Stalvey & Associates, Inc., 1140 Connecticut Ave., N.W., Washington, D.C. 20036.

6. *Journal American Medical Association:* Occasional articles of nutritional importance. American Medical Association, 536 North Dearborn, Chicago, Ill. 60610.

7. *Biodynamics:* Devoted to better farming for better health. Biodynamics, Farming & Gardening Association, Inc., R.R. 1, Stroudsburg, Pennsylvania 18360.

8. *Let's Live:* A "prestige" magazine devoted to better health for the layman. Oxford Industries, Inc., 444 North Larchmont Blvd., Los Angeles, California 90004.

9. *The Miller Message:* Very comprehensive technical review of aspects of nutritional literature. Miller Pharmacal Co., P.O. Box 229, West Chicago, Illinois 60185.

10. *Natural Food and Farming:* Better farming for better health. Natural Food Associates, P.O. Box 210, Atlanta, Texas 75551.

11. *Organicville Newsletter:* Bi-monthly informal chat on nutritional information. Organic-Ville, 4177 W. 34th St., Los Angeles, California 90005.

12. *Rodale's Health Bulletin:* Current nutritional events. Rodale Press, Inc., Emmaus, Pennsylvania 18049.

13. *Prevention:* Health and better health by prevention. Rodale Press, Inc., Emmaus, Pennsylvania 18049.

14. *The Summary:* Shute Foundation for Medical Research, London, Ontario, Canada.

15. *Applied Trophology:* Standard Process Labs., 2023 West Wisconsin Avenue, Milwaukee, Wisconsin 53201.

The following books may be ordered through book stores or found in health stores. For a few, I will list a special source, but don't be surprised to find them "out of print," which is a polite way of saying they have been banned because they were too hot for the competition. The following authors are not the only reliable ones but they will get you started and will refer you to other sources you will wish to follow up. I have listed them alphabetically, not in order of importance nor by subject. I have omitted publishers too, since many are now in paperback.

E.M. Abrahamson, M.D. and A.W. Pezet, *Body, Mind and Sugar.* One of the earliest texts on hypoglycemia.

Franklin Bicknell, M.D. and Frederick Prescott, M.D., *The Vitamins in Medicine.* An invaluable textbook and reference.

Herbert Bailey, *Vitamin E: Your Key to a Healthy Heart,* with a foreword by Miles H. Robinson, M.D. The suppressed record of vitamin E.

Emanuel Cheraskin, M.D., D.M.D., W.M. Ringsdorf Jr., D.M.D., M.S., and J.W. Clark, D.D.S., *Diet and Disease;* also *New Hope For Incurable Diseases.*

Linda A. Clark, M.A., *Stay Young Longer;* also *Get Well Naturally;* and *Secrets of Health and Beauty* (contains some recent important nutritional research).

Adelle Davis, M.S., *Let's Eat Right to Keep Fit;* also *Let's Have Healthy Children;* and *Let's Get Well* (a superb reference book on nutritional research findings on specific diseases); and *Let's Cook It Right* (a nutritional cookbook).

John M. Ellis, M.D., *The Doctor Who Looked at Hands* (a fascinating story of vitamin B$_6$).

Catharyn Elwood, *Feel Like a Million* (contains excellent laboratory nutritional research findings).

Dr. Carlton Fredericks and Herbert Bailey, *Food Facts and Fallacies.*

Dr. Carlton Fredericks and Herman Goodman, *Low Blood Sugar and You.*

Walter B. Guy, M.D., *Chemistry in Therapeutics* (out of print — the chemistry of acid-base balance).

Beatrice Trum Hunter, *Consumer Beware!* and *The Natural Foods Cook Book.*

W. Jennings Isobel, M.R.C.U.S. (University College, Cambridge University, England), *Vitamins in Endocrine Metabolism* (Charles R. Thomas, Springfield, Illinois).

D.C. Jarvis, M.D., *Arthritis and Folk Medicine.*

Royal Lee, D.D.S. and William A. Hanson, *Protomorphology*** (a textbook on protomorphogens).

W. Coda Martin, M.D., *A Matter of Life* (a blueprint for a healthy family).

Sir Robert McCarrison, M.D., *Studies in Deficiency Disease*** (with photographs — invaluable and informative); *Nutrition and Health* (with H.M. Sinclair, M.D. — available from Faber and Faber,

Ltd., 24 Russell Square, London).

Lester M. Morrison, M.D., *The Low Fat Way to Health and Longer Life* (a deceiving title for an excellent overall book on nutrition).

Weston A. Price, M.S., D.D.S., F.A.C.D., *Nutrition and Physical Degeneration* (a survey of worldwide tribes correlating diet and health with photographs). A MUST! Available through the International College of Applied Nutrition.

Sam E. Roberts, M.D., *Ear, Nose and Throat Dysfunctions due to Deficiencies and Imbalances;* and *Exhaustion: Causes and Treatment.*

Wilfrid E. Shute, B.A., M.D. with Harold J. Taub, *Vitamin E for Ailing and Healthy Hearts.*

G.M. Thienell, *My Battle with Low Blood Sugar.* (Exposition-Banner Books)

"Three Years on HCl Therapy"** as recorded in *Medical World* (a must for understanding acid-base problems).

Roger J. Williams, *You Are Extraordinary* (an approach to nutrition through anatomy). Excellent.

H. Curtis Wood, Jr., M.D., *Overfed but Undernourished* (banned at last report).

**Try to procure these books from Lee Foundation for Nutritional Research, Milwaukee, Wisconsin 53201. This foundation has been so mercilously persecuted they are almost afraid to answer letters, but try.

CHAPTER X

HOW I DIAGNOSE AND TREAT HYPOGLYCEMIA

IN MY OPINION, an examination which has 500 different check points is more valid than one which has only 100 check points. My approach is a complete metabolic examination which includes many check points.

It is easy to take short cuts and sometimes they may even prove fairly accurate. For hypoglycemia, some merely require a complete blood count, a protein bound iodine and a glucose tolerance test. If moderate control or manipulation of the patient is the aim, such evaluations are logical. If the aim is cure or as near a cure as possible, then such an examination is a farce. The patient must be understood as thoroughly as possible if cure is to be attained. Organized medicine may see absolutely no value in the extensive patient evaluation of this type but, believe me, after experience with thousands of cases it is invaluable in both the detection of hypoglycemia as well as the practice of metabolic nutritional therapy.

The routine used in my office for the complete metabolic evaluation is as follows: The patient is first expected to complete a questionnaire of some 300 questions plus making a statement of his present illness. (See Chart #1A and 1B.) There is nothing magical about the questions. After studying the answers on several different patients, patterns became obvious which give the examiner insight. This questionnaire is carefully evaluated by the examiner and the chief complaints are spelled out in detail. The patient is given plenty of time to verbalize. A dietary history, occupation and residence history as well as childhood and past histories are elicited. (See Chart 1C.) The patient is then subjected to a complete physical examination. (See Chart 1D.) Some say that it is the most comprehensive examination they have ever experienced, even though they may have had one recently prior to major surgery in a medical center.

The functional heart tests performed include the routine electrocardiogram, the phonocardiogram and pulsogram. The first test records changes in electrical potential which cause the heart to beat. The latter tests simply record heart tones and pulse waves on paper so that exacting studies can be done on heart functions. These tracings are much more exact than when the pulse is felt by the fingers or heart heard by the ear. Also, they are available for detailed comparisons at a later date.

The laboratory examination of the patient includes many different tests on the blood and urine. They are performed in a world-renowned medical testing laboratory. These tests are:

Blood

Serum glutamic oxalacetic transaminase (SGO-T)
Lactic dehydrogenase (LDH)
Total protein
Total protein with A/G Ratio
Alkaline phosphatase
Blood urea nitrogen (BUN)
Total Bilirubin
Creatinine
Glucose

Triglycerides
Lipids, total
Uric acid
Complete blood count, including RBC morphology, RBC,
    hematocrit, WBC, differential
Calcium, serum
Chlorides, serum
Phosphorus, serum
Sodium, serum
Potassium, serum
Cholesterol
Cholesterol esters
Phospholipids/Cholesterol ratio (PL/C)
Protein bound iodine
T4
VDRL
Protein fractionation
Thymol turbidity
Prothrombin time
Febrile agglutinations: rheumatoid arthritis, infectious
                      mononucleosis, Typhoid H and O,
                      Paratyphoid A and B and Proteus OX

Urine

Urinalysis, complete routine
Chlorides
Melanin
Calcium
Phosphorus
Potassium
Sodium
Uric acid
Urea nitrogen

The mineral evaluation of hair is another test, comparatively new, which is processed in a laboratory specializing in mineral analyses. The sodium, potassium, calcium, magnesium, manganese, iron, copper, zinc, lead, mercury, lithium, and cobalt are now almost routinely studied via hair analysis. It is amazing what information is derived from these tests. The

ALAN H. NITTLER, M.D.
1830 COMMERCIAL WAY
SANTA CRUZ, CALIFORNIA 95060

CASE NO.

NAME: (LAST) _____ (FIRST) _____

ADDRESS: _____ TELEPHONE No. _____ / _____ DATE _____

REFFERRED
BY: _____ S.S. No _____ BIRTH DATE ___ / ___ / ___

MARITAL STATUS
S-M-W-D x _____ YEARS _____

In your own words, what are your chief complaints? Onset, duration, severity, current status.

1.

2.

3.

4.

5.

6.

INSTRUCTIONS: Check the symptoms that apply to you. Use x, xx, xxx. xxxx, to indicate severity of the problem. Answer **ONLY** if symptoms apply to your case. Please note whether problem is present, past, or both.

Past	Now		Past	Now		Past	Now	
		Abnormal craving for sweets			Bookworm			Crave salt
		or snacks			Bottle fed			Crave sweets
		Abnormal thirst			Bowel movements painful			Crawling sensation of skin
		Acid foods upset			Breathing irregular			Cries easily for no reason
		Acne			Brittle fingernails			Cuts heal slowly
		Adencids			Brown spots or bronzing			Damp weather bothers
		Afternoon headaches			of skin			Dandruff
		Afternoon "yawner"			Bruise easily "black and			Dark glasses
		Aging rapidly			blue" spots			Day dreamer
		Air swallower			Burning feet			Daytime sleepiness
		Alcohol consumption			Burning or itching anus			Decreased amount of urine
		Allergies—tendency to asthma			Burning on urination			Decrease in appetite
		Aluminum cooking utensils			Burning stomach sensations.			Dental caries
		Ankles swell in evening			eating relieves			Depressed
		Ankles swell in morning			"Butterfly" stomach, cramps			Difficulty swallowing
		Appetite excessive			Can't decide easily			Digestion rapid
		Appetite reduced			Can't gain weight			Dizziness
		Armed forces			Can't start in a.m. before coffee			Drinks _____ cups coffee daily
		Arthritic tendencies			Can't work under pressure			Dry mouth—eyes—nose
		Aspirin history			Cataracts			Dry or scaly skin
		Awaken after few hours sleep			Chemical or spray poisoning			Drug reaction
		—hard to get back to sleep			Chemicals in environment			Dull pain in chest or radiating
		Aware of "breathing heavily"			Chronic fatigue			to left arm, worse on exertion
		Bad breath (halitosis)			Cigarette cough			Dwell on past
		Bad dreams			Circulation poor, sensitive			Eat often or get hunger pains
		Bifocals or trifocals			to cold			or faintness
		Billiousness			Cloudy urine			Eat rapidly
		Bitter, metallic taste in mouth			Coated tongue			Eat slowly
		in mornings			Cold sweats often			Eat when nervous
		Black stools			Color blind			Egotist
		Bleeding gums			Constipation common			Electrocardiogram history
		Bloating of intestines			Constipation, diarrhea			Eyelids and face twitch
		Blood in stool			alternating			Eyelids swollen, puffy
		Blurred vision			Convulsions			Eyes blink often
		Blushes easily			Crave candy or coffee in			Eyes blur after meals
		Body order bad (B.O.)			in afternoons			Eyes bulge

CHART 1A

Past	Now	
	Eyes or nose watery	
	Eye strain	
	Exhaustion—muscular and nervous	
	Extremities cold, clammy	
	Fainting spells	
	Faintness if meals delayed	
	Falling hair excessive	
	Fasting history	
	Fatigue easily	
	Fatigue, eating relieves	
	Fearful	
	Fever easily raised	
	Fluorescent lighting	
	Fluoridated toothpaste	
	Fluoridated water	
	Flush easily	
	Food "faddist"	
	Food-poisoning history	
	Frequency of urination	
	Fussy	
	Gag easily	
	Gagging reflex slow	
	Gas shortly after eating	
	Gets "drowsy" often	
	Get "shaky" if hungry	
	Glasses	
	"Going crazy" sensation	
	Gooseflesh common	
	Gooseflesh seldom	
	Greasy food intolerance	
	Gum chewer	
	Hair coarse, falls out	
	Hair treatments, sprays, etc.	
	Hallucinations	
	Hands and feet go to sleep easily, numbness	
	Hand tremor	
	Hard to awaken	
	Hate criticism	
	Headaches	
	Headaches upon arising— wears off during day	
	Heart palpitates for no reason	
	Heart palpitates when hungry	
	Hiccoughs frequently	
	High altitude discomfort	
	Highly emotional	
	History of gallbladder attacks or stones	
	Hoarseness frequent	
	Hunger between meals	
	Impaired hearing	
	Increased amount of urine	
	Increased appetite	
	Increased blood pressure	
	Increased sugar tolerance	
	Increased frequency of urination	
	Increase in weight	
	Indigestion—½ to 1 hour after eating	
	Indigestion—3 to 4 hours after eating	

Past	Now	
	Kidney trouble	
	Lack energy	
	Laxatives used often	
	Laxatives—kind used	
	Left handed	
	Light colored stools	
	Loses temper easily	
	Loss of taste for meat	
	Loud talker	
	Low back pain; flank	
	Low blood pressure	
	Lower bowel gas several hours after eating	
	"Lump" in throat	
	Malocclusion	
	Magnifies insignificant events	
	Mentally alert, quick	
	Mental sluggishness	
	Milk drinker	
	Moods of depression, "blues" or melancholy	
	Mucous colitis	
	Muscle cramps, worse during exercise; get "charley horses"	
	Muscle—leg-toe cramps at night	
	Muscle twitching	
	Nails split	
	Nails weak, ridged	
	Nausea	
	Nerve pains	
	Nervousness	
	"Nervous" stomach	
	Night sweats—cold	
	Night sweats—hot	
	Noises in head, or "ringing" in ears"	
	"Nose bleeds" frequent	
	Opens windows in closed room	
	Orphaned early	
	Overeating sweets upset	
	Overexertion reactions	
	Overwork	
	Pain between shoulder blades	
	Perfectionist	
	Perspiration increase	
	Perspiration decrease	
	Perspires easily	
	Photophobia	
	Poor memory	
	Pulse fast at rest	
	Pulse slow, irregular	
	Pulse speeds after meal	
	Pyorrhea	
	Reduced initiative	
	Respiratory disorders	
	Ringing in ears	
	Saccharin and/or sweeteners	
	Schemer	
	Sensitive to cold	
	Sensitive to hot weather	
	Sex desire increased	
	Sex desire reduced or lacking	
	Shortness of breath on exertion	

Past	Now	
	Stiff neck	
	Stomach "bloating" after eating	
	Stool floats in bowl	
	Stool has foul odor	
	Stools alternate from soft to watery	
	Strong light irritates	
	Stuffy nose	
	Sty history	
	Subject to colds, asthma, bronchitis, bronchiectosis	
	Sunburns easily	
	Susceptible to colds	
	Swallowing difficult	
	Take drugs	
	Take vitamins	
	Talk little	
	Teflon cooking utensils	
	Tendency to anemia	
	Tendency to hives	
	Tendency to ulcers, colitis	
	Tension under the breastbone, or feeling of "tightness"—worse on exertion	
	Thin, moist skin	
	Tobacco user ...... how much	
	Tremor	
	TV at home or work	
	TV color	
	Urine bubbles in bowl	
	Vomiting frequent	
	Walk with difficulty in dark	
	Weakness after colds, influenza	
	Weakness, dizziness	
	Weight gain around hips or waist	
	Worrier, feel insecure	
	Wrist watch rash	
	X-rays	

FEMALE ONLY

Past	Now	
	Age menses started	
	Days of flow	
	Period interval	
	Last period	
	Facial hair	
	Very easily fatigued	
	Premenstrual tension	
	Painful menses	
	Depressed feelings before menstruation	
	Menstruation excessive and prolonged	
	Painful breasts	
	Menstruate too frequently	
	Vaginal discharge	
	Surgical menopause	
	Menopausal hot flashes, etc.	
	Menses scanty or missed	
	Acne, worse at menses	
	Melancholia of long standing	
	The Pill	

MALE ONLY

CHART 1B

Indoor occupation	Sigh frequently, "air hunger"	Urination difficult or dribbling
Smoky urine	Skin peels on soles of feet	Prostate trouble
Insomnia	Skin rashes frequent	Night urination frequent
Intestinal trouble	Sleepy after meals	Melancholia
Intolerance to heat	Sleepy during day	Pain on inside of legs or heels
Inward trembling	Slow pulse, below 65	Feeling of incomplete bowel
Irritable and restless	Sluggish nerves	evacuation
Irritable: annoyed easily	Smelly urine	Lack of energy
Irritable before meals	Sneezing attacks	Migrating aches and pains
Itching skin and feet	Soft water	Tire too easily
Joint stiffness in evening	Sour stomach frequently	Avoid activity
Joint stiffness in morning	Special dislikes	Leg nervousness at night
Keyed up—fail to calm	Spraying in house or garden	Diminished sex desires
Kidney stones	Staring—blinking reduced	Painful urination

I hereby give my permission and consent that my case records may be used for research and educational purposes.

Patient's Signature: _____ Date _____, 19____

FOR DOCTOR'S USE: PAST HISTORY

Rheumatic Fever	Mumps	Exercise pattern	Syphilis	Hearing Loss
Cardiac	Scarlet Fever	Allergy	Gonorrhea	Goiter
Cancer	Small Pox	Jaundice	Polio	Chemical poisoning
Tuberculosis	Whooping Cough	Nephritis	Meningitis	Skin problems
Asthma	Chicken Pox	Malaria	Diabetes	Obesity
Drug reactions	Bronchitis	Typhoid	Arthritis	Emotional problems
Measles	Pneumonia	Diptheria	Epilepsy	Sleep pattern

OCCUPATION—Details _____

Past 24-hour **Food Intake:** Breakfast _____

Lunch: _____ Snacks: _____

Supper: _____

SURGICAL HISTORY: (date and kind) _____

Obstetrical History: _____

Accidents and injuries: _____ Religion: _____

FAMILY HISTORY:
(IF DECEASED, AGE AT DEATH AND CAUSE)

HOFFER-OSMOND DIAGNOSTIC TEST REPORTS

Date										
T S										
Per S										
P S										
D S										
R S										
F S										

FATHER: AGE_____ HEALTH_____

MOTHER: AGE_____ HEALTH_____

BROTHERS AGE_____ HEALTH_____

AGE_____ HEALTH_____

SISTERS: AGE_____ HEALTH_____

AGE_____ HEALTH_____

HISTORY OF: (IN WHOM)

CANCER _____

GOUT _____

ALLERGY _____

TUBERCULOSIS _____

GOITER _____

OBESITY _____

INSANITY _____

DIABETES _____

NEPHRITIS _____

HEART DISEASE _____

EPILEPSY _____

OTHER _____

CHART 1C

FOR DOCTOR'S USE

PHYSICAL EXAMINATION:

		SITTING		RECUMBENT		STANDING	
TEMP_____ PULSE_____ RESP_____		BP-RT_____ LT_____		BP-RT_____ LT_____		BP-RT_____ LT_____	

HT_____ WT_____ GENERAL APPEARANCE: _____

SKIN _____ MUCOUS MEMBRANE _____

EYES: VISION_____ PUPIL_____ EOM_____ SCLERA_____ ARCUS SENILIS RT_____ LT_____

EARS: HEARING: RT_____ LT_____ WAX: RT_____ LT_____ DRUMS: RT_____ LT_____

MOUTH: BREATH_____ TEETH: UPPER_____ LOWER_____ GUMS_____ GENERAL_____

   TONGUE: COLOR_____ TREMOR_____ EDEMA_____ FISSURES_____ PAPILLARY ATROPHY_____ PROTRUSION_____ COATING_____

NOSE:_____ LIPS:_____ THROAT:_____ PHARYNX_____ TONSILS_____

NECK: CAROTIDS: RT_____ LT_____ MOBILITY_____ OTHER_____ THYROID_____ A.R.T_____

CHEST: SYMMETRY_____ MOTION_____ SHAPE_____ BREASTS_____

HEART: _____

LUNGS: _____

ABDOMEN: _____ HERNIA: RT_____ LT_____

RECTUM: _____ PROSTATE: SIZE_____ CONSISTENCY_____

PELVIC: _____

EXTREMITIES: LEGS: RT_____ LT_____ ARMS: RT_____ LT_____

BACK: _____ RUGOFF SIGN: RT_____ LT_____

LYMPHATICS AND NODES: CERVICAL_____ INGUINAL_____ OTHER_____

REMARKS: 1 _____

2. _____

3. _____

4. _____

5. _____

6. _____

7. _____

8. _____

9. _____

10. _____

11. _____

12. _____

13. _____

14. _____

15. _____

REFLEXES:

ELECTROCARDIOGRAM: _____

PHONOCARDIOGRAM: _____

PULSOGRAM: _____

H-O DIAGNOSTIC TEST: _____

35MM SLIDE STUDY: _____

LABORATORY: _____

ROUTINE PANEL: _____

PAP SMEAR: _____

HAIR: _____

OTHER: _____

NUTRITIONAL PROGRAM: _____

AHN 870

CHART 1D

blood tells only what is in the blood with no regard as to whether the substance is coming or going. The urine registers the excretion or going. The hair, however, does register what is happening on the cellular or orthomolecular level. I have found this extremely valuable in the practice of nutritional therapy.

The patient is also asked to get a five-hour, seven-specimen glucose tolerance test from a hospital or laboratory of his choice but according to my directions.

We also perform the HOD test. This is the Hoffer-Osmond Diagnostic Test. It is a simple card test perfected to determine the patient's emotional pattern.

Finally, there is evaluation by means of photographs. The patient is photographed with a special camera so that physical details can be recorded. The patient is routinely examined in full view from the four sides. The mouth is recorded with the lips closed, the mouth open, the teeth exposed, the gums, the tongue out and under the tongue. The pair of eyes is photographed from a medium distance and individual eyes from a close-up view. The palms, dorsums and backs of the hands are photographed. So are the feet and any other part of the body which seems to be unusual, such as rashes, moles, bruises, discolorations, deformities, etc.

A week later, when laboratory tests are available, the findings of the examination are discussed with the patient, except the hair analysis, which takes another week or two, and a program is set up for the patient. The details are explained. All this is recorded on cassette tape and given to the patient so that he can refer to the discussion and directions at home as often as he desires.

Glucose Tolerance Test

The five- or six-hour glucose tolerance test is the

backbone for making the diagnosis of hypoglycemia. There must be a specimen taken at the first half hour as well as at the start and at each hour of the test. In my estimation, the test should be taken after a simple twelve-hour fast without any other special dietary preparations. Some feel that the patient should stuff on carbohydrates for three days prior to the test. I do not believe that this is fair to the patient. It makes him sick before the test is run, thus insuring an abnormal test result.

Here again there is a temptation for short cuts. Some doctors think that a simple three-hour test is sufficient. As pointed out previously, many hypoglycemic conditions do not come to the fore before the fourth or even fifth hour. Some believe fasting, plus a one-hour test, is enough to make the diagnosis. While it is true in some cases, yet if this scanning test is normal, which it is many times, the whole test must be done anyway. To me there is no substitute for the real thing: the five- or six-hour test with the first one-half hour specimen taken along with the hourly ones.

Knowing which test is being used by the laboratory is necessary for proper evaluation. The Folin-Wu test with a normal fasting range of 80-120 mgm% is a good test. So is the true blood sugar test with a normal fasting range of 60-90 or 70-110 mgm%. It makes no difference in interpretation which test is being used so long as its identity is known.

Criteria of Interpretation of the Glucose Tolerance Test

There are five criteria which have been set up as standards of normalcy. They are as follows:

1. The blood sugar level must rise to the half hour thence on up to the one hour level.

2. There must be no more than a minus 20% differential between the fasting and the lowest levels. (NOTE: This may be a bit strict because some authorities feel that a minus 5% differential is significant.)
3. There must be no level below the normal low point for the fasting specimen.
4. The drop from the highest point to the lowest point should be about 50 mgm%.
5. The one-hour level must be at least 50% more than the fasting level.

When these five criteria are routinely applied to the evaluation of the five-hour, seven-specimen glucose tolerance tests, one begins to see the true dynamics of hypoglycemia. It is my opinion that hypoglycemia can be diagnosed even if only one criterion is abnormal. One must beware of a false sense of security if the curve seems to be close to normal. In my experience a near normal test does not necessarily indicate a lesser severity of hypoglycemia than a test which is further from normal. The test curve gives no reliable indication as to type or severity of the clinical status.

Many times the criteria presented here can be misused in relation to the diabetic. In the diabetic, the early hour values are extremely high and do not return to fasting levels until after the two hour mark. Even so, the drop from the high point to the low may easily and usually does exceed the 50 mgm% criterion of #4. (The drop from the highest point to the lowest point should be about 50 mgm%.) Therefore, one qualification to the above criteria must be that the glucose not remain at elevated levels too long. If the high or diabetic level falls to a very low level in the later hours, then the diagnosis is dysinsulinism. Dysinsulinism is a combination of hyper- and hypoglycemia. The patient is diabetic at one point only to become hypoglycemic shortly thereafter. This causes many problems in treatment if the low levels are ignored and the patient is treated only for diabetes.

Dynamics of Glucose Tolerance Test

In my opinion the actual numbers involved in the glucose tolerance test are not so important as the dynamics of the test. By this I mean how high, how low, how fast and how precipitously the changes become the important factors. This makes the test a dynamic one rather than a simple routine of numbers.

Therapy

The correct therapeutic approach to hypoglycemia demands the proper attitude on the part of the physician. There is a multiple aim which includes adequate intake of nutrients, proper digestion, optimal preparation for metabolism (liver function), satisfactory delivery to the tissues (good cardiovascular system), normal metabolism and good excretion. All of these vital functions must be normal before body harmony exists. When harmony exists, there is no illness and the patient is well. The aim of therapy is to normalize the vital functions. The effort of the physician to attain harmony is of primary importance.

The proper attitude of the physician at this stage of knowledge concerning hypoglycemia should be rated good, better and best. His goal should be nothing but the best. It is necessary to be unprejudiced. There is much bickering in the profession about food quality, food supplements and use of the adrenocortical injection. Some organized medical experts persist in recommending sugar to overcome the symptoms of low blood sugar. Sugar merely gets the patient out of one crisis only to throw him into another. Sugar is the basic evil in the tale of woe for the hypoglycemic. Other doctors use tranquilizers, ACTH or corticosteroids. I am absolutely against the use of the corticosteroids and ACTH. The tranquilizers do have one redeeming feature: they buy time. Unfortunately, tranquilizers frequently are used as continued treatment when they should only be used as a temporary measure.

Intravenous glucose can be a life-saving type of therapy under certain circumstances. It certainly is neither curative nor does it last more than just a few hours. In fact, in the case of blood sugar fluctuations, what goes up must come down: glucose aggravates hypoglycemia.

Various Approaches

One very obvious conclusion regarding therapy for hypoglycemia is that there is no drug which gives a real or lasting result. If a satisfactory drug were available, organized medicine would be head over heels in treating hypoglycemia. Surgery is not the answer for the same reason.

The first breakthrough of any significance was made by Seale Harris, M.D. with his dietary approach. This was a big step because it combined causative factors with the therapeutic treatment. Later, John Tintera, M.D. combined the stress adaption syndrome of Hans Selye, M.D. to the dietary approach of Harris, thus taking the next real therapeutic step. Diet plus supplementary nutrition had been my approach prior to my contact with Dr. Tintera. My approach at present is diet plus injections plus supplementation. Organized medicine still only offers surgery, psychotherapy, tranquilizers and sugar as therapeutic methods.

The dietary approach can be merely a modified normal diet recommendation where one is told not to eat carbohydrate and to eat protein. Other diets can be a bit more sophisticated in that specific quality of the foods is specified. For example, raw foods in preference to cooked foods or butter in preference to oleomargarine. Diets can also be aimed at detoxification.

My particular dietary approach is what I call the Target Diet. During the first two weeks the patient is to follow a mono or duo diet as listed. (See Chart 2.) The diet is to be this same food for two weeks. It is not a hodge-podge of single food meals. The intake should be eight times daily to be sure that the blood sugar is held at relatively constant levels. During the second two weeks the diet is to be restricted to areas 10 and 9 in the target area. (See Chart 3.) This allows a reasonable increase in the intake but is still quite restrictive compared to a so-called average diet. The third two week interval is to be restricted to 90% in areas 9 and 10 and 10% in area 8. (See Chart 4.) Again, an increase in varieties of foods. The final two weeks are to be 80% in areas 9 and 10 and 20% in area 8. Thus we have four different levels of dietary intake corresponding to the degree of detoxification and the capability of the patient's digestion. This dietary regime covers the first eight weeks of my therapeutic program. Area 7 of the Target Diet is the "Never-Never" land in the world of malnutrition. (See Chart 5.) Unfortunately, this represents the customary American diet. Thus, I am condemning the usual American diet. Many of my patients tell me that due to this program they have been awakened to a new and better way of life and will never return to the old.

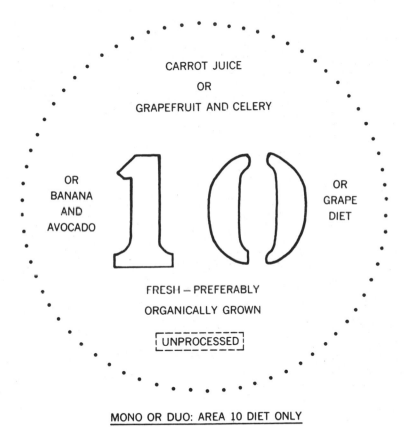

CARROT JUICE

OR

GRAPEFRUIT AND CELERY

OR
BANANA
AND
AVOCADO

OR
GRAPE
DIET

FRESH – PREFERABLY
ORGANICALLY GROWN

UNPROCESSED

MONO OR DUO: AREA 10 DIET ONLY

CHART 2

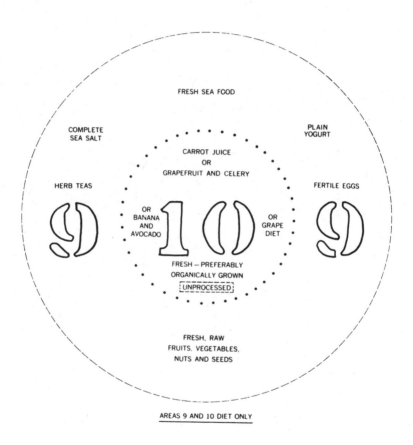

FRESH SEA FOOD

COMPLETE
SEA SALT

PLAIN
YOGURT

CARROT JUICE
OR
GRAPEFRUIT AND CELERY

HERB TEAS

FERTILE EGGS

OR
BANANA
AND
AVOCADO

1 O

OR
GRAPE
DIET

FRESH — PREFERABLY
ORGANICALLY GROWN
UNPROCESSED

FRESH, RAW
FRUITS, VEGETABLES,
NUTS AND SEEDS

AREAS 9 AND 10 DIET ONLY

CHART 3

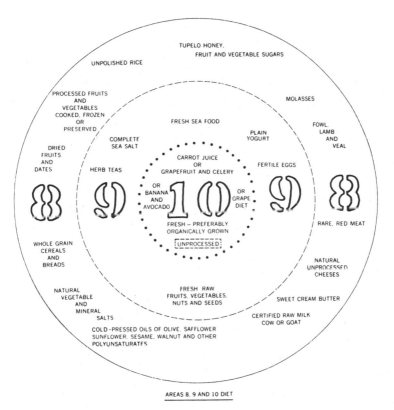

AREAS 8, 9 AND 10 DIET

CHART 4

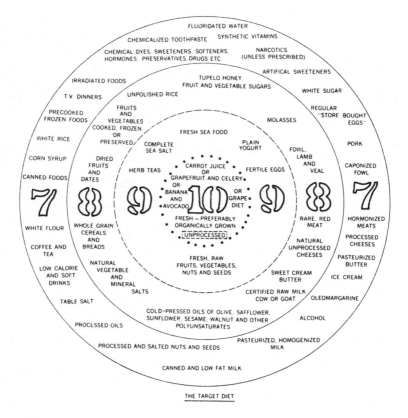

THE TARGET DIET

CHART 5

Injections

One of the two major injection procedures is the administration of adrenocortical extract (ACE) in oil. This is the whole adrenal cortex gland extract. It is not related to cortisone except that it is rated in terms of cortisone. All the hormones secreted by the adrenal cortex glands are present in ratios as they occur naturally. One of these thirty-odd hormones is cortisone. They are naturally balanced and thus cannot cause an artificial imbalance of the hormone system as that caused, for instance, by cortisone. Whole adrenocortical extract is *not* the same as cortisone nor does it have the same action! Under no situation is one part equal to the whole.

The ACE in oil injection acts in the system for about 30 hours. It tends to suppress function of the adrenal cortex glands by becoming a substitute for them. It is, therefore, important to develop a preconceived plan as to phasing out this injection before the patient becomes accustomed to it. My usual plan is to give the patient an injection three times weekly for the first month, twice weekly the next month and then once weekly for the third month. This takes him up to the three month point which will be discussed later. ACE in oil is administered intramuscularly. I consider the oil ACE program somewhat inferior to the aqueous ACE program. Dosage is 0.9 cc per injection.

The other approach is to use the aqueous adrenocortical extract (aqueous ACE). Again, this is not cortisone. *It is the whole adrenocortical extract.* The usual plan of action is to give the injection intravenously once weekly for three months. Sometimes, when symptoms or stresses are very great, more frequent injections are given in the early stages of treatment in order to get better and quicker results for the patient. Injections may even be given daily for limited periods. Actually, 90 percent of the patients achieve very satisfactory results in twelve weeks' time on the once weekly schedule. Some of the 10 percent get good results in up to twenty weeks or less.

My favorite intravenous injection consists of the following:

a. Aqueous adrenocortical extract   1000 mcgm
b. Vitamin B-12 (cyanocobalamine)   1000 mcgm
c. Vitamin C (ascorbic acid)   250 mg
d. Vitamin B-6 (pyridoxine)   100 mg
e. Calcium glycerophosphate   2 cc
    (Calphosan .®)
f. Dilute Hydrochloric acid 1:1000   10 cc

Naturally, either of these two methods of injections is combined with the dietary approach. If one must make a choice between the use of the injections or the diet and supplements, I always recommend the latter because the curative power of the program exists in correct diet and supplementation. The injection is merely the catalyst to speed the reaction.

After the three-month intensive nutritional therapeutic period, the patient usually feels greatly improved. When the injections are combined with the dietary and supplemental program results are faster. This three-month period with injections equals the degree of improvement usually achieved by the patient in 18 to 24 months or more without the injection. These figures apply to an estimated nine out of ten patients. The effects of the intravenous injection last about four hours. This four-hour period, when combined with the detoxifying mono or duo diet plan, gives the patient an adrenocortical rest period wherein his body can attempt to rebuild itself. Weekly injections allow time for tissue regeneration between injections.

Nutritional Supplements

My whole nutritional supplement program is based upon liver detoxification. This is spelled out in detail in Chart 6. This chart represents an eight-week period. At the top, one can see the four two-week periods in the various dietary phases. Under this are a series of products listed in the week in which they are to be started or changed in dosage. For instance, the first week, the patient is to start the Betaris, Choline, Cholacol II and Hepatrophin. The next week other items are to be started while the first week items are continued. Two Betaris are given eight times daily in the second and third weeks, reverting to two four times daily the fourth week, and so forth.

Upon this basic liver detoxification plan the individual patient program is built. These added items represent the need of each patient gleaned from the history, physical examination and the various laboratory and functional tests. It is an highly individualized program.

Concerning vitamins, I attest that *all* vitamins are essential for life and good health. The therapeutic philosophy is to prescribe them all in abundant quantity. The body can choose what and how much it needs for repair purposes if all are present. Sometimes, if extra large dosages of a certain vitamin are needed, different products will be prescribed so that the body has the best chance of utilizing what is needed from several sources.

An attempt is also made to provide an intake of all the minerals, whether gross or trace, in abundant quantities. Inorganic and organic minerals

Basic Program For:

Date:

WEEK 1	2	3	4	5	6	7	8	MAINTENANCE
100% Area 10 Diet, 8 meals per day		100% Areas 10 & 9 Diet, 8 meals per day		90% Areas 10 & 9 Diet, 10% Areas 8—6 meals per day		80% Areas 10 & 9 Diet, 20% Areas 8—5 meals per day		
THINK THIN		CHEW THOROUGHLY				EAT SLOWLY		

Betaris 2-4 x daily
Choline 1-3 x daily
Cholacol II 4 before meals—1 x daily
Hepatrophin 1-3 x daily
Catalyn 1-3 x daily
Minoplex 1-3 x daily
Cal-Amo 1-3 x daily

Betaris 2-8 x daily
Chlorophyll Complex 1-3 x daily
Betalco 1 daily
Cataplex C 1-3 x daily

Betaris 2-4 x daily
1-2 x daily
Protefryn 1 daily
Zypan 1-3 x daily
Antronex 1-3 x daily
Cataplex B 1-3 x daily
Cataplex G 1-3 x daily

Cholacol 1-3 x daily
1-2 x daily
Soy Bean Lecithin 2-3 x daily

1-3 x daily
Renatrophin 1-3 x daily
Zymex II 1-3 x daily

NOTE: Substitute products are not the same. The patient must be under his personal physician's observation during detoxification period. Bring this form with you when you visit your physician.

No 571—AHN

ALAN H. NITTLER, M.D.
1830 COMMERCIAL WAY   PHONE (408) 4754111
SANTA CRUZ, CALIFORNIA 95060

CHART 6

are both important. Usually there are special needs in each case.

Regarding types of minerals, there are a couple of necessary principles to understand. Soluble vs. insoluble characteristics are important. On one hand we have sodium chloride, which is quite soluble, and barium sulfate, which is insoluble. Both are inorganic compounds. On the other hand, there is cider vinegar vs. kelp. They are respectively soluble and insoluble in the organic realm. Another principle to consider is the organic vs. the inorganic. Chlorophyll is soluble and organic; magnesium sulfate, soluble and inorganic though both are types of magnesium compounds. Adequate nutrition includes all combinations of organic, inorganic, soluble and insoluble mineral forms.

A third type of mineral compound is relatively new and known as "chelated." It is not truly organic as formed in nature but is "man-made organic." Man takes certain desired minerals and combines them with predetermined desired organic compounds. These chelated compounds are a kind of in-between substance theoretically having the better qualities of each. Laboratory studies show that chelated minerals are assimilated up to three times more efficiently than inorganic minerals.

The cytotrophins or protomorphogens are used at the orthomolecular nutritional level to improve utilization of all vitamins and minerals used in the program. The cytotrophins taken directly from specific organ sources are used to stimulate liver and kidney function as well as actions of heart, pancreas, adrenal, brain and other human organs. The various cytotrophins are used as need is determined. The comprehensive aim is to detoxify and to rebuild the tissues at the same time.

There are some digestive aids which enhance the nutritional program. Acidophilus yeast is one of great value. The type of intestinal flora influences the status of health of the body. The acidophilus yeast is very conducive to the development of the friendly bacteria. I consider the acidophilus yeast better in establishing friendly flora in the intestinal tract than the acidophilus bacteria; the yeast is more sturdy than the bacteria. An adequacy of hydrochloric acid and pepsin in the stomach is also a *must* for good digestion. This is frequently overlooked and antacids erroneously given instead because the symptoms of too much and too little acid can be practically identical. Pancreatic enzymes and bile salts in abundance enhance digestion. *Comfrey-Pepsin* clears the intestinal tract for better assimilation.

How does one measure results in patient care? One thing we should *not* do is to ask the physician himself! His answers are always prejudiced. The real answer is forthcoming from the patients. They are the ones who know the results first hand. Patients are extremely critical. However, it is necessary to obtain this patient information in some objective way. They are human, too, and do not necessarily remember correctly the exact status as of a year or two ago. To bypass this, I repeat the use of the questionnaire and analytic program as done originally. I also use the before-and-after photographic technique, to provide a more objective means of evaluation.

Another point in evaluation is the time element. In my program there are the eight week, twelve week, six month and twelve month points of evaluation. One can expect different but definite improvement results at the various points of evaluation.

It is more realistic to talk about the degree of control because once a hypoglycemic, always a hypoglycemic. There seems to be no real escape from this. I will state positively, however, that the degree of control of hypoglycemia is very satisfactory in the great majority of my patients. Approximately 90 percent are greatly improved. I wish every one of you could talk to my patients.

CHAPTER XI

MEDICAL CASE HISTORIES

MALNUTRITION IS a factor in every illness. It is the only one, aside from stress, of the major etiological factors of disease which can be significantly controlled. Nutritional deficiencies can cause general or local areas of malnutrition. Local malnutrition results in abnormal function of the cells and tissues involved and opens the door to disease. Disease usually does not attack normal tissues; local tissue function must be imbalanced before disease can set in. Therefore, malnutrition predisposes to disease.

Nutritional Method

The aim of the nutritional method is to discover, correct and rebuild these involved tissues. The whole body is involved, therefore it must be an overall approach. When the metabolic malfunction has deteriorated sufficiently structural damage can result. In order to insure the process of healing, there must be a restoration of the nutrients in tissues. Building up a reserve supply of nutrients also fortifies the body in times of stress.

Nutritional improvements or corrections occur at different rates depending upon the tissues involved, the intensity of the deficiency, and the degree of corrective effort. There are constant adjustments and readjustments in metabolic function as well as in healing. Therefore, symptoms vary from day to day. Some days are better than others during the overall improvement period.

Nutrition for the Practitioner

The remainder of this book is dedicated to the medical practitioners, as they practice their specialty. It is meant to be a stimulus for understanding and application of some nutritional truths to their own practices. For illustrative purposes, I have chosen a few cases from my files.

The usual medical approach to a case is discussed only superficially. There is no attempt to deny the value of drug therapy. The purpose is to demonstrate that there is another approach which is an additional spoke in the wheel of therapeutics. It is simply a matter of adding the "thinking nutritionally" attitude toward every problem.

Ultimate success is to utilize *all therapeutic methods* in varying degrees in each case, depending upon need. This is where the practice of medicine really is tested. Remember the importance of the nutritional factors of disease first, because they are of major importance. When additional help is needed, even drugs and surgical techniques can be used more successfully together with a positive nutritional treatment program. Good nutrition cannot hurt the patient during any type or stage of therapy. It can only be an asset.

Products

Brand names are used in this book because of the nature of their quality. Quality in many products is usually neither designated nor protected by labels. The only safeguard in evaluating which products are dependable is the reputation of the manufacturer. Just because certain substances are allowed legally is no guarantee that they are effective nutritionally.

There is no such thing as a chemical equivalent to natural supplements.

Companies whose products are valuable in my practice are:

1. *Natura Brand, Inc.*, M.F.R., Moonachie, New Jersey 07074
2. *Seroyd Brands, Inc.*, P.O. Box 125, Lafayette, Calif. 94549
3. *Standard Process Laboratories*, 2023 West Wisconsin Ave., Milwaukee, Wisconsin 53201
4. *Sunshine Valley*, 8725 Remmet, Canoga Park, Calif. 91304
5. *Viobin Corp.*, Monticello, Illinois 61856
6. *Vitamin Products Company*, 2023 West Wisconsin Ave., Milwaukee, Wisconsin 53201
7. *Westpro Laboratories*, 12975 Main St., Garden Grove, Calif. 92640

Other brands may be good even though I am not familiar with them. However, in all my experiences, I have never found something that is "just as good as" the original. Copies are never of the same quality. In nutritional therapy, product quality is a must! Lack of quality is sometimes the reason why some practitioners are unsuccessful with nutritional therapy. It certainly delayed my progress at times. Since the results may not be forthcoming as anticipated, the whole concept may be tossed out the window as a farce. I again emphasize that in order to get desired responses, be sure to use the best products available. Take the word of one who has done it; then, after you have experience, you may do some experimentation on your own. When you know first hand what can be accomplished nutritionally, there will be no holding you back in your own search.

Here are a few case histories, written in the patients' own words, followed by my medical notes and the therapy I used in each case.

CASE HISTORY I: Housewife

"I hardly know where to start in expressing my extreme gratitude for your program of treatment for me.

"When I came to you I suffered from swelling and tingling of extremities, almost constant hunger, periodic weakness, great sensitivity to glare and to loud noise. I felt the need to sleep following a meal and experienced excessive bleeding and fatigue during my menstrual periods.

"Since becoming your patient I find myself energetic and alert until nearly midnight, awake fully by around 7:30 or 8 each morning, in good spirits, not sluggish, and continuing throughout the day glad to be alive, performing challenging tasks. Only very rarely have I felt a need to sleep during the day—and this only when I have stayed up excessively late the previous night or when I have undergone extreme emotional tension.

"Previously I drank large amounts of coffee in a vain attempt to raise my lagging, absent energy. After a cup or two—or more—I would very briefly feel livelier—and then would come a lower slump. I would perhaps eat a candy bar or indulge my near-addiction to spaghetti or white bread or cereal. No wonder I weighed as much as I did! A seesawing of mood accompanied my hypoglycemic physical pattern.

"Never have I felt weak or hungry while on the diet you have prescribed for me. During this time I have not once departed from the diet and do not intend to, as my joy in feeling really well for the first time in my life far outweighs the momentary satisfaction of a taste thrill of former days. Actually I enjoy all of the fine foods permissible. I have discovered new taste delights in the variety of natural foods. I no longer crave the empty calories I previously consumed daily. Needless to say I feel more comfortable, more agile, and more attractive physically as well as in a better frame of mind when I see a new slimmer me in passing a window or mirror and when dressing for the day.

"Our entire family is benefiting from the wisdom of your care. I find friends asking, 'Isn't it hard to cook for the rest of the family and not eat the food yourself?' My answer is No. I do not prepare for my family what I now know to be unnutritious. We eat only health-promoting foods. We buy only fertile eggs, raw certified milk, whole grain, stone ground bread, real butter. I feel that our present diet, though seemingly more expensive, is not actually so, since we do not waste our money on the empty calories and harmful foods we previously purchased. Our desserts of fresh fruit, dates, nuts, our large fresh salads are all taste treats as well as body builders. Finally we are investing our food dollar squarely where it belongs — in our health.

"As I write this I look up occasionally and out of our window at the ocean — with no dark glasses, no strain, no squint . . . a new experience for me.

"Before I became your patient I had visited several skin specialists in the hope of finding help in the removal of what appeared to be growths on my face. Biopsies were taken; result negative. I asked how to get rid of these growths; how to prevent their growing back. I received a shrug of the specialist's shoulder (later, his bill!); he didn't know! Dr. Nittler took one look at the area involved and prescribed medication for external application which within one week's time cleared up the difficulty. It has not returned.

"I had become discouraged in past years not only with the methods of more orthodox medical men in terms of what I felt to be inadequate testing before diagnosis, but also with the side effects of drugs administered so readily and so abundantly. On one occasion in particular I recall having received treatment for what the throat specialist mistakenly diagnosed (without lab test) as an *infection:* potent drugs, various drugs—over a three-month period. Many dollars poorer and weakened from all these drugs, some of which provoked severe allergic reaction, I went on my own to a lab. The diagnosis: pellagra, a *deficiency* disease. It had apparently not occurred to the specialist to suspect diet as a causative factor, to realize that in nutrition lay the key to my case.

"Dr. Nittler's scrupulous care in administering exhaustive tests and his prescribing in terms of those results for each individual patient impress me most favorably. I have the greatest confidence in Dr. Nittler's understanding of *my* health picture—its needs, assets, liabilities, the balancing of my body chemistry —as well as his concern for my personal well-being in every way. He is always patient in answering my questions about myself or another member of my family. I value Dr. Nittler's character and integrity. I feel him to be honest, dedicated, and highly skilled in his specialty of metabolic nutrition. Daily I see evidence of the value of his treatment of me. The benefits of Dr. Nittler's detoxification program began to be apparent almost at once. As the months go by, I find that this new-found good health is being sustained and even increased."

Medical Report

This 45-year-old well-developed, obese white female first consulted me on 4-8-70 at which time complaints of swollen ankles and overweight were made. She was tired of taking thyroid 1 grain daily, estrogen 1.25 mg. daily along with a diuretic. Her past history revealed the usual childhood diseases without complications, infectious mononucleosis in 1965, mild hay fever and allergic reaction to penicillin. She was a secretary and housewife. She used white bread, jelly, saccharin and margarine in her usual diet. At age six she had had a double mastoidectomy and a subtotal thyroidectomy in 1954. She had delivered three children, without complications, who were living and well. Family history showed a father who had had cancer and tuberculosis, mother with colitis, allergies, obesity and nephritis.

The physical examination revealed a well-developed, obese white female who was 5'6-1/2" tall and weighed 180 pounds. She was alert, cooperative and pleasant. The temperature was 98.8° and pulse 90 reg. BP Sitting R 115/90 L 120/80 Recumbent R 120/-90 L 95/80 Standing L 100/80. Skin had + petechiae. Eyes were normal except for + + congestion of the sclera. Ears were normal. Mouth was negative except for + + gold caps and + + amalgum fillings. Tongue was + red, + tremor and + coated. Nose, throat, lips and pharynx were normal. Tonsils were out. Neck was negative except for an ART (achilles reflex time) reaction of 260 milliseconds which demonstrated a slightly hypothyroid (euthyroid hypothyroidism) condition. Chest was normal and the breasts were very large but without mass or tenderness. Heart was regular and without murmur or rub and was not enlarged. Lungs were clear to percussion and auscultation. Abdomen was + + + + obese and without masses but was + + tender throughout the course of the colon. Pelvic examination showed a normal multipara with a normal cervix, normal adnexae. The legs revealed some small venules which were dilated.

Routine laboratory work revealed the following positive findings: Urine: High phosphorus of 1.34 gm/24 hrs., low sodium 1.86 gm/24 hrs., chlorides low at 4.6 gm/24 hrs. Blood alkaline phosphatase slightly high. White blood count 12,200. Differential segs-67, bands-3, L-24, E-0, B-0, M-6. A five hour glucose tolerance test of 96-168-116-102-88-68. Normal fasting range 70-110. The Pap smear was Class I, normal and the maturation index was 0-30-70. (Normal 0-15-85)

The electrocardiogram was normal. The pulsogram did not reveal arteriosclerosis. The pulse wave was very small and corresponded to that of a 3-1/2 year old child. The character was ill defined. The phonocardiogram was distorted in several ways revealing need for nutritional support. Summary: no heart disease but functional insufficiency secondary to malnutrition. The HOD test was normal concerning emotional problems.

Therapeutic Program

She was started on a basic liver detoxification program with added emphasis on heart, bone marrow, thymus, thyroid, ovary, uterus and adrenal glands. These structures needed special support as gleaned from the history and physical examinations. She was also given extra minerals and vitamins containing the naturally associated synergistic factors. Her skin problem responded to a Standard Process product known as USF (unsaturated fatty acid ointment). In addition, she was given the intravenous injection designed to aid and abet the adrenal cortices.

After a few weeks, her improvement was obvious. She blossomed out with energy in all facets of life. Her weight dropped to 159 even though I do not consider this a primary weight reducing program. Her blood pressure remained normal or even dropped a little which is quite common on this program. This has been a very excellent response and one that makes all the other trials worthwhile.

CASE HISTORY II: Male Dentist

"Three years previous to the time I presented myself for treatment in Dr. Nittler's office I was diagnosed as hypoglycemic by a local physician who had carefully performed an extensive and thorough examination. My chief complaint at that time was extreme hunger and weakness 4-1/2 hours after meals. This physician advised that I eat carbohydrates such as candy, doughnuts or sweet rolls upon onset of hunger symptoms for relief — which I did for a time and then discontinued and trained myself to put up with the symptoms. Gradually the symptoms increased and there were others that became apparent. These were insomnia, nervousness, extreme fatigue, difficulty to concentrate, anxiety, numbness in legs and dread of work.

"For several years I would have four or five hours of uninterrupted sleep and then little or no sleep the rest of the night. The local physician prescribed an hypnotic drug for sleeping, saying to use it only when necessary and not to abuse its use. I would usually take one sleeping pill every five or six days for rest and then would feel much better for two or three days, then the poor sleeping pattern would return. The fatigue that I experienced would become more pronounced each succeeding day until I would again have a good night's sleep after taking a sleeping pill. For added energy I would have two or three cups of coffee for breakfast and also at lunch time.

"The nervousness and anxiety that I experienced

seemed to vary in indirect proportion to the amount of sleep. During periods of nervousness and anxiety I would have difficulty in concentrating and would frequently postpone making decisions in routine office procedures until I could logically reason them through. After a time the practice of dentistry, which I had always enjoyed, became a drag. I actually dreaded the thought of going to work and would look forward to leaving the office.

"My legs became intermittently numb for two years and then were numb most of the time for a year prior to seeing Dr. Nittler. This was something I accepted and tried to live with.

"Golf had been my favorite avocation for the past twenty years. During the last two or three years I steadily lost interest in the game. I experienced anxiety and nervousness when I would play golf. I would find myself worrying because I didn't play better and would also feel depressed after playing. After a year of this routine I stopped playing golf almost completely.

"Now after one year's treatment by Dr. Nittler all of the symptoms mentioned have either diminished or disappeared completely. I have followed the prescribed treatment plan completely, I am sleeping better, I am enjoying my work and look forward to going to my office in the morning. I feel my attitude in general is much improved and I again have a sense of well being."

Medical Report

Dr. O., a 49-year-old dentist first came to me 8-7-70 complaining of lack of energy, difficulty in sleeping and occasional nervousness. The lack of energy had been present for 4-5 years and was getting worse. The insomnia had been present for about ten years and consisted of awakening early with the inability to get back to sleep. By early, he meant about 2-3 A.M. He also did not go to bed until around ten or eleven, so he was getting very little sleep. The nervousness was primarily when he was working under pressure. His past history was relatively noncontributory except that he contracted mumps encephalitis in his teens and had a residual transient stiff neck. He also suffered from hay fever for many years. Being a Seventh Day Adventist, he was on a relatively good diet except that he was drinking coffee with cream and sugar. This was about six or more cupfuls per day. (Note: coffee except when used as an enema is harmful, particularly to hypoglycemics.) He had an appendectomy in 1938 without complications and a T & A in early childhood. He was the father of two children, one of whom had died accidentally at age nine. There was no history of accidents or injuries. His entire family history was noncontributory.

The examination revealed a well-developed, well-nourished 49-year-old white male of approximately the stated age. He was alert, cooperative and pleasant. T-97 P-80 reg. BP Sitting R 135/90 L 120/90 Recumbent R 120/80 L 130/80 Standing L 140/100. He was 5'11-1/2" and weighed 175 pounds. Skin was with + + petechiae and red moles. Eyes were corrected with bifocals, pupils were equal, round and reacted to light and accommodation, extra ocular movements were full but with a fine bilateral nystagmus, sclera were + congested and mucous membranes were normal. Ears contained + wax but were considered well within normal range. Mouth: breath OK. Teeth were repaired with + + + gold inlays, gums OK and general health of mouth was good. Tongue was + pale + tremor + edema + fissures + + papillary atrophy, protrusion OK and

+ coated. Nose, lips, throat, and pharynx were OK. Tonsils out. Neck negative for nodes and thyroid swelling, achilles reflex time 270 milliseconds (high normal indicating borderline hypothyroidism). Chest was normal. Heart was regular and without murmur or rub and was not enlarged. Lungs were clear to percussion and auscultation. Abdomen was soft and without mass or tenderness. He had + + bilateral Rogoff's sign (pressure tenderness in costo-vertebral angle) indicating adrenal tenderness. Peripheral reflexes were abnormal in that the biceps and knee jerks were absent bilaterally. The HOD test showed normal emotional balance.

Laboratory work was extensive and only the positive findings are recorded here: Urine: specific gravity was low, 1.009, phosphorus high, 1.7, uric acid high, 1.0. Blood: all routine chemistries were normal. The five-hour seven-specimen glucose tolerance with normal fasting range 70-100 test was: 79-100-85-50-60-69-83 which is a very low and flat curve indicating poor glucose metabolism.

His electrocardiogram was normal except for a splintered QRS V-3 Elevated S-T in V-3, V-4, V-5, and a slightly inverted T-aVL. Heartogram or pulsogram showed no evidence of arteriosclerosis, a variable pulse wave in consecutive beats and diminished volume of the pulse wave which indicated a weakness of heart function from the nutritional angle. The phonocardiogram revealed poor balance between first and second tones, poor quality of tones as compared to normal standards, variable sequential tones, excessive exercise response and general evidence of weak stamina due to nutritional deficiency.

Therapeutic Program

He was started on a basic detoxification and rebuilding program consisting of enzymatic support, protein rebuilding, glandular stimulation along with vitamin and mineral supplementation. He was also started on the intravenous aqueous ACE mixture injection for adrenocortical support. The injections were given for three months at weekly intervals as was the supplemental program in its maximum form. After the three months of intensive nutritional therapeutic effort, the therapeutic program was gradually reduced toward a maintenance level. At one year he visits the office on a quarterly basis for discussion and perhaps an injection and is on a maintenance supplemental program.

His clinical response has been very satisfactory. He is able to work full time with the normal amount of energy, sleep well, even seven to eight hours at a time. He can even nap while watching TV before retiring and still sleep all night. He has control of his life even under pressure and manages a full dental practice which he enjoys.

CASE HISTORY III: Young Woman

"I am a woman of 29 years of age. I have always been a person who wanted to do as many things as possible but I have never had the energy or stamina or a strong constitution. As a child, I was small and thin and I did not like athletics. It always hurt too much, and I exhausted quickly. I had to have many enemas because of constipation. Laxatives were routine. I can still vividly conjure up the taste of castor oil—ugh!

"When I was in high school, I had a barium enema X-ray which determined there was nothing actually wrong with my bowels. I just had a lazy peristalsis action. My periods were bad and laid me up for three days each time. Many times I had violent cramps and vomiting, and a sensitive stomach. No one told me this could have been due to not having bowel movements more than once or twice a month. I assumed it was period time (which was so irregular I could not tell).

"I was married at eighteen and had my first baby at nineteen. I started on a round of bladder, vaginitis and kidney infections. Every time I was given antibiotics to control the bladder problems I would get a vaginitis infection. I was told by many doctors that there was no connection. My gynecologist thought there was. He sent me to several specialists. I wound up in a university hospital for a week where I had a proctoscopy and a cystoscopy. It was discovered my ureters were too long and kinked like a garden hose where the infections of my kidneys and bladder began. I was sent home and told to drink from one to two gallons of water a day for the rest of my life and was given a stool softener with instructions to use as needed.

"During this period of my life, fatigue was 'normal.' I became pregnant again during which time I had never felt better although I was still constantly tired. In 1967 my husband and I were divorced and I went to work. They sent me to a psychiatric clinic because they believed my problems were psychosomatic. I marvel that I made it through the next two years—they were rough. In 1969 I remarried, and for the first time in my life was allowed the luxury to be sick. My body went on a strike and I wanted to sleep all the time. My headaches got worse and worse although there was now no emotional foundation for them.

"What finally sent me back to a doctor was another kidney infection. A friend recommended Dr. Nittler. I had been told a couple of years before that I 'probably had hypoglycemia' although no tests were given to me by the doctor. He had told me to eat something every two hours or so. When I was working I ate sweets—doughnuts and candy bars and sweetened coffee—to keep from getting dizzy.

"I went to see Dr. Nittler January 23, 1970. Following his diet and vitamin prescriptions, my headaches stopped. There is a note in my journal on February 4th—'Headache is gone!' I started having regular bowel movements. They are now daily or multiple daily! My attitudes are happier—life is worth living. I have even been able to make it through the day without a nap. Believe me, to wake up in the early morning and have the energy to be able to listen to the birds sing is a joyful experience. I give thanks for another day of living."

Medical Report

This 29-year-old white female first consulted me on 1-23-70 with the complaints of kidney problems of many years duration for which she was finally advised to drink 1-2 gallons of water per day (even worse, she was drinking fluoridated water!). She suffered from headaches, lack of energy, low grade fever, backaches, leg swelling, aches in hip joints, deep cough with retching when exposed to cold air and infrequent bowel movements. She thought it was normal to have one or two movements per month. All these complaints seem to have been present most, if not all, of her life. In her past history we find that she had the usual childhood diseases without known complications. She had pneumonia in 1966 without complications. There was a question in her mind as to whether she had nephritis and diabetes. She suffered frequently from a recurrent vaginitis.

Her dietary for the previous twenty-four hours was horrible according to my standards. There was bread, jam, oleo, coffee and not enough fresh vegetables and fruit. Her surgical history consisted only of having had a cystoscopic examination at which time she was determined to have a kinked ureter. She had delivered two children 6-1/4 and 9-1/2 years previously. She was currently taking the Pill. She had suffered a back injury during high school age.

Her family history contributed only to the fact that there were two members of the family who had suffered from diabetes: mother and grandfather.

Physical examination revealed a well-developed white female who appeared well-nourished. T 98.0 pulse 70 reg. BP Sitting R 110/80 L 110/80 Recumbent R 120/85 L 120/85 Standing L 130/80. She stood at 5'4-1/2" and weighed 141-1/4 pounds. Skin was clear. Eyes with good vision, pupils equal, round and react to light and accommodation, extraocular movements full and regular, sclera + congested and the mucus membranes OK. Ears were OK for hearing, + + wax in the canals and the drums were not visualized. Mouth: + strong breath, + + + amalgum fillings, gums OK and general health of mouth, fair. Tongue was + pale, 0 tremor, + edema, + papillary atrophy, protrusion OK and + + coated. The nose, lips, throat and pharynx were normal and the tonsils were atrophic. Neck was normal and the ART was 240 milliseconds (midnormal). Chest was symmetrical with good motion and normal shape. Breasts were large and without mass or tenderness. Heart was regular and without murmur or rub and was not enlarged. Lungs were clear to percussion and auscultation. Abdomen was + + obese and + + tender in right upper and lower quadrants. The cervix was inflamed and had some cysts on it which were cauterized. The fundus was in antero-position and the adnexae were negative. The dorsal spine was grossly malaligned. Condition of extremities not remarkable and the reflexes physiological.

The positive laboratory findings were: Urine: low sodium of 2.7 grm/24 hrs. and a low chloride of 6.0 gm/24 hrs. The Pap smear was Class I negative and maturation index was 0-95-5 (norm 0-15-85). Blood: VDRL neg., differential count was Bds. 8, Segs-75, L-13, E-0, B-0, M-4. The five-hour seven-specimen glucose tolerance test was 95-145-140-90-110-55-80 with a normal fasting range of 80-120. The electrocardiogram was entirely within normal limits. The pulsogram did not demonstrate arteriosclerosis and was of good character except that the volume of the pulse curve was a little low. The phonocardiogram showed a three tone beat in the aortic and mitral areas. The heart tone ratios were abnormal and sequential tones were, for the most part, similar. The exercise response was within normal range. These latter two tests showed the need for nutritional support to the heart. The HOD test was normal and did not reveal any emotional abnormality.

Therapeutic Program

She was started on a basic detoxification program with extra nutritional supplement support for the heart, kidneys, adrenals, pituitary, ovaries, bones and spleen. Her special program was developed upon a basic liver detoxification plan. She was also given the intravenous ACE injection on a weekly basis for 16 weeks since she had a stormy time with detoxification and had a recurrence of the cystitis during the program period. She then was on the two-week injection interval for seven months and then abruptly to the one-month interval. The usual program routine was altered because of her slow response to therapy. The supplemental intake was also reduced at these mentioned points. I anticipate a time when these can be cut considerably more as she demonstrates that she can get along well without so much support. She also had one bout of pneumonia at the fourteen-month point but managed not to get so sick as usual and remained ill for a shorter time. Her stamina certainly has improved.

CHAPTER XII

NUTRITIONAL THERAPY FOR THE SPECIALIST

THE FOLLOWING DISCUSSION covers various ailments routinely referred to various specialists. I have described the nutritional therapy which has proven successful in my experience. I present these methods for your serious consideration.

Allergist: Asthma

I. *General Discussion:*
   A disease marked by recurrent attacks of paroxysmal dyspnea, with wheezing, cough, and a sense of constriction, due to spasmodic contraction of the bronchi. The paroxysms last from a few minutes to several days: they may result from direct irritation of the bronchial mucous membrane or from reflex irritation. Many cases of asthma are allergic manifestations in sensitized persons.

II. *Nutritional Considerations*
   A. Physiological review:
      1. Predisposing factors: Malnutrition, low carbohydrate tolerance, adrenal insufficiency, stress situations, gastrointestinal disorders, congenital predisposition.
      2. *Associated entities:* Skin diseases, hypoglycemia, hypotension, colitis, chronic indigestion, lowered resistance, alkalosis, allergies.

3. *Common clinical manifestations:* Emotional instability, metabolic disturbances (adrenal, pituitary, etc.), catarrh, sinusitis, hay fever and other allergic manifestations.
4. *Special physiological considerations:* The older the patient, the more intractable. In infancy, most likely a food allergy. In children, poor nutrition and general run-down condition. In adults associated with gastrointestinal involvements.

III. *Nutritional Therapeutic Approach:*

Catalyn	— Basics
Drenaplex	— Adrenal hormone precessors
Pneumatrophin	— Relieves lung congestion; specific cell stimulator
Antronex	— Anti-histamine effect; liver hormone
Cataplex C	— Increases O_2 carrying capacity of blood protein protective factors
Cataplex E	— Increases O_2 utilization ratio
Cataplex A	— Normalizes mucous membrane activity
Betalco	— Liver metabolism factors
Calcium Lactate	— Diffusible calcium
Comfrey-Pepsin, Betaine HCL in adults	— Improves digestion
Wheat germ oil perles for children	— Improves cell respiration

Thymus for treatment
in infancy   — Abets antibody
                                formation
SPECIAL: Vitamin A & C   — Desensitizer
  Cataplex A-F Betaris   — Liver decongestant
  Zymex   — Intestinal detoxicant

Cardiologist: Arrhythmia

I. *General Discussion*
   Abnormal heart rhythm: auricular fibrillation,
   atrial flutter, premature ventricular contractions,
   tachycardia, heart block, pulsus alternans.
II. *Nutritional Considerations*
   A. Physiological review:
      1. *Predisposing factors:* Malnutrition, rheu-
         matic heart disease history, hypertension,
         hyperthyroidism, enlarged heart.
      2. *Associated entities:* Neuritides, malnutri-
         tion, short of breath, ankle edema, muscle
         twitching, excessive use of tea, coffee, to-
         bacco, hypoglycemia.
      3. *Common clinical manifestations:* Fainting,
         syncopal attacks, weakness, congestion of
         lungs, gastric or cerebral symptoms, dis-
         tention of jugular veins.
      4. *Special physiological considerations:*
         Adaption to sudden changes in rhythm of
         heart difficult. One step closer to death
         than if arrhythmia did not exist — a vital
         situation. Symptoms a result of deficiency
         therefore correct deficiency immediately
         to relieve symptoms and the gravity of the
         situation. If the condition is cured before
         the cardiologist is consulted, which fre-
         quently happens, the impression is that
         the condition did not exist in the first
         place.

III. *Nutritional Therapeutic Approach:*

Catalyn	—General Support
Cardiotrophin	—A heart extract to regulate metabolism of heart muscle fibers
Cataplex E	—Manganese and phospholipid metabolism (nerve sheaths)
Cataplex G	—Enzyme precursor factors for proper cholinesterase action
Cataplex C	—Increase O_2 carrying capacity of blood
Cataplex B	—Lactic and pyruvic acids metabolism; improve motor nerve conductivity
Cataplex E-2	—Phospholipid synergist of alpha tocopheral to conserve O_2
Cataplex F	—Calcium diffuser
Phosphade	—Reduce blood viscosity; autonomic nervous system factor
Calcium Lactate	—Improves muscle tonicity, ionizable calcium
Wheat germ oil perles	—Antioxidant
Allorganic trace minerals	—Potassium source; trace minerals source

Many other and various supplements are used for specific and individual needs.

Dentist: Caries

I. *General Discussion:*

Caries is the molecular decay or death of a bone, in which it becomes softened, discolored, and porous. It produces a chronic inflammation of the periosteum and surrounding tissues, and forms a cold abscess filled with a cheesy, fetid, puslike liquid, which generally burrows through the soft parts until it opens externally by a sinus or fistula. Dental caries is a disease of the calcified tissues of the teeth resulting from the action of micro-organisms on carbohydrates characterized by a decalcification of the inorganic portions of the tooth and accompanied or followed by disintegration of the organic portion. It is of four degrees of severity: caries of first degree, in which the enamel alone has become decalcified; caries of the second degree, in which the enamel and dentin are affected; caries of the third degree, in which the pulp is exposed; caries of the fourth degree, in which the pulp has undergone putrefactive degeneration.

II. *Nutritional Considerations:*

A. Physiological review:

1. *Predisposing factors:* Sticky, sweet foods; colas; mineral deficiency (not fluorine).

2. *Associated entities:* Malnutrition, intestinal worms, sweet tooth, affluence.

3. *Common clinical manifestations:* Gingivitis, peridontaclasia, malocclusion.

4. *Special physiological considerations:* Prevention starts with basic diet as early in life as possible, even in intrauterine life— raw, uncooked and non-pasteurized foods. A refined and cooked food disease only found when demineralized and devitaminized foods are used.

III. *Nutritional Therapeutic Approach:*

Bio-Dent	—Biologically active veal bone calcium-protein-enzyme factors
Cataplex F	—Calcium diffusing factors
Calcium Lactate	—Diffusible calcium
Cataplex ACP	—Connective tissue factors
Minaplex	—Potassium and alkaline ash minerals
Ostogen	—Bone cytotrophin— uncooked veal bone— protein-mineral-complex (determinant)
Acidophilus Yeast	—Improves intestinal environment for better absorption
Zypan	—Gastric secretion catalyst; cooperates with acidophilus yeast
Catalyn	—General nutrient support

Dermatologist: Psoriasis

I. *General Discussion:*
A chronic, recurrent papulosquamous dermatosis, the distinctive lesion being a silvery gray scaling papula or plaque. Lesions form serpiginous areas; dull pink or red color, sharply defined, somewhat elevated, surrounded by healthy skin, covered by dry, poorly overlapping scales which are readily detached. Hair unaffected. Skin beneath is dry and slightly excoriated. Nails become dry, lusterless and whitish; become raised and separated from bed and may be partially or completely lost.

II. *Nutritional Considerations:*
A. Physiological review:
1. *Predisposing factors:* Disturbances in fat

metabolism, biliary sluggishness.
2. *Associated entities:* Malnutrition, allergies, peripheral arteriosclerosis, hypoglycemia.
3. *Common clinical manifestations:* Dry, scaly skin.
4. *Special physiological considerations:* Pork could be principal offender by allergic reaction.

III. *Nutritional Therapeutic Approach*

Cataplex A-F Betaris	—Lowers bile viscosity; decongestion of liver; cholesterol elimination
Zypan	—Improves digestion; gastric enzyme catalyst
Betalco	—Liver metabolism factors
Cataplex G	—Cell proliferating factor; fat metabolizing factors
Cataplex E	—Increases tissue response to stress
Thymex	—Phagocytosis and lymphatic drainage factors
Phosphade	—Lowers blood viscosity; gland accelerator
Vitamin A & C (urea)	—Desensitizing factor; osmotic transfer of tissue fluids
Soy Bean Lecithin	—Fat transporter; cholesterol antagonist

General Practitioner: Dizziness

I. *General Discussion:*
A disturbed sense of relationship to space; a sensation of uncertainty or unsteadiness in the head with a feeling of movement within the head not associated with movement of objects or uncoor-

dination. Usually disappears when the individual is recumbent. It may be constant or transient. Dizziness is to be distinguished from vertigo which is a sensation as if the external world were revolving around the patient.

II. *Nutritional Considerations:*
   A. Physiological review:
      1. *Predisposing factors:* Quite variable when due to vegetative disorders, treatment depends upon correction of cause. High blood pressure due to high cholesterol and poor cerebral circulation with compensation by the increased blood pressure. Packed cerumen against the ear drum. Calcified ossicles and blocked Eustachian tube. Anemia.
      2. *Associated entities:* Ménière's syndrome. Liver overload with more carbohydrate and fat ingested than can be assimilated. Malnutrition, low blood volume secondary to diarrhea, vomiting, hemorrhage, etc. Intracellular vs. extracellular fluid balance disturbances; shock, etc. Hypoglycemia. Mineral (electrolyte) deficiencies.
      3. *Common clinical manifestations:* Neurasthenia, acidosis (cannot hold breath longer than 20 seconds), mineral depletion (need salt), motion sickness and hyperventilation syndrome.
      4. *Special physiological considerations:* Common symptom, associated with many different clinical entities.

III. *Nutritional Therapeutic Approach*
   Catalyn —General nutritional factors
   Neurotrophin —Specific cell activator

Cal Amo	—Combats respiratory alkalosis
Cataplex F	—Calcium diffuser
Niacinamide—B-6	—Vasodilator, liver metabolism
Phosphade	—Gland accelerator factor; lower blood viscosity
Solar dried sea or earth salt	—Trace mineral replacement
Seromins	—Chelated mineral source
Cataplex B	—Support nerve tissue
Vitamin A & C	—Urea source
Eustachian tube manipulation (Muncie technique)*	—Equalization of atmospheric pressure

Gynecologist: Amenorrhea

I. *General Discussion*
Absence or abnormal stoppage of the menses. Normal state: prepuberty, postmenopausal, during pregnancy, the puerperium and the lactation periods. Occurs after double oophorectomy, hysterectomy or after radiation therapy.

II. *Nutritional Considerations*
A. Physiological review:
1. *Predisposing factors:* Anemia (hypochlorhydria), endocrine insufficiency, metabolic changes (thyroid, climate, work, mental stress, overwork, worry).

---

*Dr. Douglas Muncie. D.O., 150 N.E. 96th St., Miami, Fla. 33138 or 1940 E. Charleston, Las Vegas, Nev. 89014.

2. *Associated entities:* Malnutrition, hypoglycemia, chronic debilitating diseases: Tuberculosis, diabetes, nephritis, oophoritis, hypothyroidism, cachexia, anemia.
3. *Common clinical manifestations:* Pallor, fatigue and other signs of anemia; subnormal nerve integrity; acute febrile diseases.
4. *Special physiological considerations:* Amenorrhea always a symptom; usually result of endocrine hypofunction which is secondary to malnutrition.

III. *Nutritional Therapeutic Approach:*

Catalyn	—General support
Utrophin	—Integrity of uterine cells
Ovatrophin	—Integrity of ovarian cells
Chlorophyll Complex Perles	—Sex hormone precursors; prothrombin factor
Denamone	—Sex hormone precursors; antioxidants
Cataplex E	—Tissue repair rate and cellular activity enhancement; better oxygen utilization
Ferroplus	—Anti-anemic factors
Thytrophin	—For hypothyroidism, dry skin
Cataplex G	—Enzymatic nerve tranquilizer

Cardioplus   —Muscle nutrition
factors; tone,
relaxant

Gynecologist: Dysmenorrhea

I. *General Discussion:*
Painful menstruation. Hypogastric pain associated with menses which may radiate throughout lower abdomen, to the back, inguinal regions and even down the thighs. Pain usually aching in character with exacerbation of griping or colicky suprapubic pain sufficiently intense to produce nausea and vomiting on occasion.

II. *Nutritional Considerations:*
 A. Physiological review:
  1. *Predisposing factors:* Loss of electrolytes: Calcium, iron, potassium via kidneys and lowered blood glucose.
  2. *Associated entities:* Malnutrition, constipation, hypoglycemia.
  3. *Common clinical manifestations:* Premenstrual weight gain, nervousness, leukorrhea, dysuria, endocrine imbalances.
  4. *Special physiological considerations:* Due to dilution of blood constituents because of compensatory edema (change in intra- and extracellular balance).

III. *Nutritional Therapeutic Approach:*

Cataplex E   —Reduces cellular oxygen demand

Calcium Lactate   —Ionizable calcium

Pituitrophin   —Endocrine mobilization

Ovatrophin   —Specific cell activator

Cataplex B   —Oxidizes lactic and pyruvic acids

Vitamin A & C (urea)	—Diuretic; osmotic transfer factor
Chlorophyll Complex Perles	—Sex hormone precursor; prothrombin factor
Catalyn	—General nutritional support
Parotid Cytotrophin	—Muscle relaxant
Seromins	—Chelated minerals or electrolyte source

Internist: Diabetes Mellitus

I. *General Discussion:*
A metabolic disorder in which the ability to oxidize carbohydrates is more or less completely lost, usually due to faulty pancreatic activity, especially of the Islets of Langerhans and consequent disturbance of normal insulin mechanism. This produces hyperglycemia with resulting glucosuria and polyuria giving symptoms of thirst, polyuria, hunger, emaciation and weakness and also imperfect combustion of fat with resulting acidosis, sometimes leading to dyspnea, lipemia, ketonuria, and finally coma. There may also be pruritis and lowered resistance to pyogenic infection.

II. *Nutritional Considerations:*
A. Physiological review:
1. *Predisposing factors:* Hereditary, malnutrition, overeating processed carbohydrate; pancreatic, islet cells, failure; zinc deficiency.
2. *Associated entities:* Arteriosclerosis: cerebral, peripheral (with gangrene), cataracts, otosclerosis, drowsiness, itching; dry mouth.

3. *Common clinical manifestations:* Gangrene and ulcerations of feet, coma, blindness-cataract, sudden amaurosis, infections and boils, polydypsia, polyphagia, polyuria, halitosis (sweet-acid type).
4. *Special physiological considerations:* Involvement of adrenals, pancreas, thyroid, liver, kidney and probably pituitary.

III. *Nutritional Therapeutic Approach:*
Exercise beneficial, muscle utilization of carbohydrate reduces need for insulin, nervous strain detrimental.

Catalyn	—General support
Pituitrophin	—Trophic control of endocrine system
Pancreatrophin	—Specific cell activator
Betalco	—Carbohydrate metabolism of liver cells
Arginex	—Kidney support factors
Cataplex B	—Lactic, pyruvic acid factor

Muscle metabolism factors:

Cardiotrophin	—Increases muscle demand for sugar
Minaplex	—Potassium ions necessary for muscle contraction
Inositol	—Phosphoralization factor
Cataplex G	—Cholinesterase precursors
Protedyn	—Completes blood amino-acid pattern; promotes transfer to tissues.

Neurologist: Headaches

I. *General Discussion:*
Pain in the head, cephalalgia. Very common complaint caused by multiple factors both localized within the cranium, in the proximal neck-shoulder area or systemic in nature. Seven basic factors of

importance: 1. location, radiation and depth; 2. duration; 3. frequency; 4. character; 5. integrity; 6. progress; and, 7. associated symptoms.

II. *Nutritional Considerations:*
   A. Physiological review:
      1. *Predisposing factors:* Sluggish cerebral circulation; muscle tension.
      2. *Associated entities:* Malnutrition, adrenal insufficiency, hypoglycemia, liver disease, spinal subluxations, dental disease.
      3. *Common clinical manifestations:* Histamine reactions, hypertension, intestinal toxins, kidney disease, eye strain, sinusitis, toxemia.

III. *Nutritional Therapeutic Approach:*

Antronex	— Antihistamine effect (not indicated in certain types of low blood pressure)
Phosphade	— Gland accelerator; lowers blood viscosity; reduces pain during attack
Prostex	— Calcium mobilizing factor
Arginex	— Systemic detoxifier by activating kidneys
Pituitrophin	— Trophic control of endocrine glands
Ruta-Plus	— Anti-capillary fragility factor
Neurotrophin	— Specific cell stimulator
Calcium Lactate	— Often aborts anticipated (aura) attack; ionizable calcium
Cataplex G	— Enzymatic antispasmodic
Orchex	— Physiological tranquilizer

Obstetrician: Pregnancy Schedule

I. *General Discussion:*
   Bearing children is one of the greatest privileges

of life. With privilege comes responsibility. Prenatal attention is as important as postnatal care. Parents should nutritionally train for parenthood starting many months before conception. The more rugged and sturdy the parents, the more likely the child will be robust. Primary malnutrition (simple deficiency) or secondary malnutrition (due to drugs, chemicals, radiation, etc.) are causes of congenital defects. Actually, specific deficiencies during gestation cause specific defects, i.e. B-6 deficiency in pregnant rats causes cleft palates.

II. *Nutritional Considerations:*
   A. Physiological review:
   1. *Predisposing factors:* Malnutrition to be avoided; super nutrition to be developed.
   2. *Associated entities:* Nausea and vomiting of pregnancy, anemia, toxemia of pregnancy, varicose veins, and hemorrhoids.
   3. *Common clinical manifestations:* Fatigue: need routine rest pattern.
   4. *Special physiological considerations:* Some researchers feel low phosphorus intake in 3rd trimester is indicated possibly because of thyroid stimulation. Evidence not convincing when raw bone meal is used.

III. *Nutritional Therapeutic Approach:*
   Plain foods high in vitamins, minerals and other nutrients. Avoid all foodless foods, synthetic foods, alcohol, cigarettes.

Catalyn	—Multiple essential food factors
Calcium Lactate	—Ionizable and diffusible calcium
Chlorophyll Complex Perles	—Sex hormone precursors; prothrombin factors

Biost	—Raw bone enzyme and amino acid factors
For Complications:	
Cal Amo	—Chloride replacement
B-6 with niacinamide	—Nausea and vomiting reduced
Ferroplus	—Antianemia
Arginex	—Kidney cleanser
Renatrophin	—Relieve kidney overload
Collinsonia	—Relieve venous congestion; liver stimulation

Ophthalmologist: Cataract

I. *General Discussion:*
An opacity of the crystalline eye lens or of its capsule.
II. *Nutritional Considerations:*
  A. Physiological review:
    1. *Predisposing factors:* Injury or shock or prolonged stress, malnutrition, congenital, drugs and chemicals, trauma, flash burn, toxemia, X-ray radiation, hereditary, calcium, cholesterol deposits. Fluorescent lighting and possibly prolonged radiation from TV.
    2. *Associated entities:* Senility, hypercholesterolemia (arcus senilis), diabetes, arteriosclerosis, hypothyroid, malnutrition, hypoglycemia, microwave oven exposure.
    3. *Common clinical manifestations:* blindness.
    4. *Special physiological considerations:* May disappear while on general nutritional pro-

gram: no specific deficiency (holistic
concept); low protein balance often present.

III. *Nutritional Therapeutic Approach:*
Extensive and slow (1/2-3 years); 50% respond.
General benefits positive even though specific
results may be a failure.

Cataplex G	—Enzymatic nerve precursor and antispasmodic factors which improve circulation
Phosphade or Biost	—Combats tissue deposits of calcium
Rutaplex	—Cholesterol metabolism
Cataplex ACP	—Connective tissue factors increase O_2 carrying capacity of blood
Oculotrophin	—Specific cell activator (when trauma or infection present, may develop histamine reaction)
Prostex	—Phosphatase source
Allorganic Trace Minerals	—Enzyme activators
Thytrophin	—Calcium/potassium ratio regulator
Pituitrophin	—Trophic control of enzymes
Eff-plus	—Phosphorus metabolizer; chromosome protector

Orthopedist: Bone Healing

I. *General Discussion:*
Healing: a process of cure; the restoration of wounded parts. After a bone fracture, all bodily forces are mobilized for bone knitting—calcium, phosphorus, protein, hormones, Vitamin D.

II. *Nutritional Considerations:*
A. Physiological review:
1. *Predisposing factors:* Age of patient, malnutrition, type of fracture: open or closed; contamination, degree of distortion; rigidity vs. flexibility of bone; strength of bones.
2. *Associated entities:* Menopause, metastases, etc.; fluorosis.
3. *Common clinical manifestations:* nonunion; cooked food disease; Paget's disease; osteomalacia, osteoporosis, hypoparathyroidism (lack calcium), avitaminosis D, hyperthyroidism, caries, disc lesions. Bone is a detoxifying mechanism; stores lead, radium, fluorine, arsenic, etc.
4. *Special physiological considerations:* Bone a living tissue; living cells alter physicochemical basis. Phosphatase necessary in healing bones (destroyed by pasteurization of milk).

III. *Nutritional Therapeutic Approach:*

Ostogen	—Specific cell activator
Prostex	—Phosphatase source
Calcium Lactate	—Ionizable and diffusable form of calcium
Minaplex	—Source of alkaline ash minerals
Eff-Plus	—Cytotrophin wrapper

Cataplex D   —Promotes absorption calcium, para-thyroid hormone

Cataplex F   —Calcium diffusing factors

Thytrophin   —Regulation calcium-phosphorus ratio

Lactic acidophilus yeast —Promotion of intestinal absorption calcium

Pediatrician and Gastroenterologist: Megacolon

1. *General Discussion:*
Abnormally large colon, due to dilatation and hypertrophy. The condition is usually one of childhood. Called also giant colon, congenital idiopathic dilatation of the colon and Hirschsprung's disease. Manifested by having one very large diameter bowel movement every 1 or 2 weeks, even up to 4 weeks occasionally. Movement commonly plugs commode.

III. *Nutritional Considerations*
   A. Physiological review:
      1. *Predisposing factors:* Improper toilet training, emotional stress, lack bulk-forming foods, liver dysfunction, hypothyroidism.
      2. *Associated entities:* Malnutrition, hypothyroidism, hypoglycemia.
      3. *Common clinical manifestations:* Constipation, toxemias, neurasthenia, intestinal putrefaction, allergies, frequent pyogenic infections, biliousness, foul breath, coated tongue, intestinal gas, bloatedness.
      '4. *Special physiological considerations:* Large, painful movements yield emotional problems; colonics (with enzymes) recommended.

III. *Nutritional Therapeutic Approach:*

Catalyn	—General support
Fleet's Phosphosoda ®	—Stimulate liver functions: physiological laxation
Thytrophin	—Promote thyroid activity
Organic Iodine	—Supports thyroid function
Drenaplex	—Promote peristalsis
Lactic acidophilus yeast	—Improve intestinal flora
Cholacol	—Cholagogue effect of bile salts
Betalco	—Liver stimulation
Hepatrophin	—Liver cell activator
Comfrey-Pepsin	—Changes bowel; supports intestinal mucosa
Betaine HCL	—Aid protein digestion

Psychiatrist: Mental Depression

I. *General Discussion:*
Anxious, agitated depression: depression felt as worry, uneasiness, agitation and panic with ideas of poverty or impending ruin.

II. *Nutritional Considerations:*
   A. Physiological review:
      1. *Predisposing factors:* Malnutrition: demineralized diets, vitamin deficiencies (B-3 and B-6). Glandular disorder: overstimulation of glands via mental stress causing mineral loss via kidneys. Aging processes: deviations in calcium metabolism: arteriosclerosis, osteoarthritis. Psychogenic: environmental factors.
      2. *Associated entities:* Hypoglycemia, hyper-

irritability, tachycardia, premature ventricular contractions, high or low blood pressure, allergies, arthritis (after climacteric), appetite changes, photophobia, dysphagia, delusions, GI problems: ulcer, colitis, diarrhea.

3. *Common clinical manifestations:* Rationalization, though acute, may be illogical; environment frequently blamed; extremes of evaluation of physical condition and personality attributes; multiple complaints; well-versed, analytical, introspective with emphasis on mental phases and tendency to omit or deprecate importance of physical nature of life.

4. *Special physiological considerations:* Demineralization; decreased O_2 reserves; B complex deficiencies.

III. *Nutritional Therapeutic Approach:*

Orchex	—Physiological tranquilizer (nondrug)
MinTran	—Mineral tranquilizer
Pituitrophin	—Trophic effects on pituitary
B Supreme	—Megavitamin therapy
Nia-Plus	—Megavitamin therapy
Cataplex B	—Water soluble B complex factors
Cataplex G	—Oil soluble B complex factors
Niacinamide—B-6	—Nerve tissue support

Psychiatrist: Insomnia

I. *General Discussion:*
Insomnia means an inability to sleep; abnormal wakefulness; inability to get proper amount of sleep. Three types: (1) inability to get to sleep, (2) awaken too early and cannot go back to sleep

and (3) repeated awakenings during night.
II. *Nutritional Considerations:*
A. Physiological review:
   1. *Predisposing factors:* Endocrine imbalances: adrenal, thyroid—low energy in A.M. high BMR at night—night owl. Emotional stress and strain, cerebral stimulation: drugs, malnutrition, vasomotor instability, liver insufficiency.
   2. *Associated entities:* Malnutrition, worry-fear-dread, senility, overindulgence in food, nocturnal leg cramps, hypoglycemia.
   3. *Common clinical manifestations:* Nightmares, hyperirritability, cramps, nocturia, toxic insomnia, anxiety neurosis, headaches, high blood pressure, allergies, manic depressive psychosis.
   4. *Special physiological considerations:* Peaceful resting, a close equivalent to sleep . . . nervous tension causes fatigue.
III. *Nutritional Therapeutic Approach:*

Catalyn	—General support
Drenaplex	—Adrenal normalizer
Minaplex	—Potassium and alkaline ash trace minerals
Licorice root tea	—Natural relaxant
Orchex	—Physiological tranquilizer
Antronex	—Liver hormone antihistamine effect
Vitamin A & C (urea)	—Denatures calcium-protein complex
Hepatrophin	—Specific cell activator
Cataplex A-F Betaris	—Decreases bile viscosity
Cataplex G	—Physiological antispasmodic
Calcium Lactate	—Ionizable calcium

Timely Tip: Retention enema using two tablespoonfuls of blackstrap molasses in one pint of water before retiring for the night may act as a very pleasant sandman.

Urologist: Benign Prostatic Hypertrophy

I. *General Discussion:*
A nonspecific benign enlargement of prostate. External growth encroaches upon rectum and causes constipation. Internal growth tends to occlude the urethra making urination difficult or impossible.

II. *Nutritional Considerations:*
  A. Physiological review:
    1. *Predisposing factors:* Aging: up to 40% of men over 60 yrs.; truck drivers, infection, male sex.
    2. *Associated entities:* Malnutrition, hypothyroidism, vitamin F and calcium metabolism, cystitis, impaired drainage.
    3. *Common clinical manifestations:* Night urination, dribbling, lose force of stream, burning sensations, low back pain, constipation, impotence, hip pain.
    4. *Special physiological considerations:* Liver dysfunction prevents proper metabolism of vitamins F-1 and F-2.

III. *Nutritional Therapeutic Approach:*

Cataplex F	—Enhance fat digestion, calcium diffuser
Prostate Cytotrophin	—Specific cell activator
Arginex	—Kidney cleanser
Calcium Lactate	—Ionizable and diffusible calcium

Chlorophyll Complex Perles	—Sex hormone precursor
Nucleo-protein	—Cell metabolism factor
Cataplex ACP	—Epithelial and connective tissue factors
Ribo-Nucleic Acid	—Cell blueprint factors
Thytrophin	—Thyroid activity synergist

Some of these nutritional concepts may be quite foreign to your thinking. They were to mine, too. It took a lot of trial and error before I accepted them. Even now. I sometimes wonder why they are working but the one thing that is outstanding is that the results are forthcoming when the substances are used as directed.

I urge you, try them for yourself before you condemn them. You could be pleasantly surprised. I hope you will join the ranks of those who have the courage to add nutrition—either gradually or completely—to your practice. And when you do, please let me know so that I can refer patients in your area to you. I have a growing number of requests for a nutritional doctor from countless patients from all over the country who wish this type of help.

Alan H. Nittler, M.D.
1830 Commercial Way
Santa Cruz, California 95060

abdomen, 158, 163, 167
absorption, 51-52
ACE (adreno-cortical extract), 57,
   82, 138, 145, 168; aqueous, 145,
   146, 164
acidophilus yeast, 45, 150, 175;
   lactic, 188, 189
ACTH, 139
Addison's disease, 63
adenoidectomies, 40
adrenal cortex glands, stress-
   caused exhaustion in, 63
adrenalin, 62, 64
adrenocortical extract, see ACE
adulterated foods, 14, 20
alcohol, 2, 60
alfalfa seed sprouts, 96
allergic tendencies, 38, 43, 53;
   asthma as manifestations of, 170
allopathic physicians, 10, 80, 115
allorganic trace minerals, 173, 186
Aloe vera plant, 105, 106
amenorrhea, 178-80
American Journal of Clinical Nutrition, 124
American Medical Association, 34;
   Journal of, 124
amino acids (protein factors), 3,
   4, 8, 47, 48
angina pectoris, 100
antacids, 93
antibiotics, 45, 104, 165
anticoagulants, 27
anti-pollution laws, 24
Antronex, 171, 183, 191
Applied Trophology, 125
Arginex, 182, 183, 185, 192
arrhythmia, 172-73
ART (achilles reflex time), 158,
   163, 167
arterial problems, 113
arthritis, 43
Arthritis and Folk Medicine by
   D.C. Jarvis, M.D., 126
ascorbic acid, 3, 146; synthetic,
   102, 105

assimilation, adequate, 13, 82
aspirin, 68, 85, 92
asthma, 170-72; nutritional aid for,
   75-76; as allergic manifestation,
   170
athlete's foot, 103-4
atomic radiation, 23-24

barium sulfate, 149
barley water, 91
bay (laurel) leaves, 106
beet-root powder, 37
benzoin compound, tincture of,
   103
beriberi, 39
Betaine HCL, 171, 189
Betalco, 171, 176, 182, 189
Betaris, 92, 147
blood count, 7, 128
blood tests, 85, 129-30, 159, 163,
   168
blood pressure, 160; high, 88
bile, flow of, 12, 92
bile salts, 51, 91, 150
Bio-Dent, 175
Biodynamics, 125
bioflavonoids, 3
Biost, 185, 186
birth control measures, hazards
   of, 25-26
body function, formalization of, by
   nutritional therapy, 4, 11, 12-14
Body, Mind and Sugar by E.M.
   Abrahamson, 55-56, 126
body parts, interrelation of, 2;
   nutritional needs of individual,
   2-4
body rub, apple cider vinegar, for
   fever, 98; for colds, 102; for
   poison oak and ivy, 106
boils, 104
bone healing, 187-88
books on nutrition therapy, 35,
   126-27
BP, 158, 162, 167
brainwashing, commercial, at ex

pense of nutritional education,
8, 15, 122. *See also* drugs and
drug industry *and* FDA
bread compress, 104
burns, 105

Cal Amo, 178, 185
calcium glycerophosphate, 146
calcium lactate, 7, 101, 102, 171,
173, 175, 180, 183, 184, 187,
191, 192
California Medical Association, 34
Calphosan, 146
cancer, 8
carbohydrates, natural, 2, 61, 86,
136, 160; man-made, 61
cardiogram, 66, 67
Cardioplus, 180
cardiotrophin, 50, 173, 182
cardiovascular system, good, 138
caries, dental, 118, 174-75
carob, 91
carotenoids, 3
castor oil, 90, 106-7, 164
Catalyn, 171, 173, 175, 177, 179,
180, 182, 184, 189, 191
Cataplex A, 102, 171; ACP, 175,
186, 193; A-F Betaris, 172, 176,
191; B, 173, 178, 180, 182, 190;
C, 50, 171, 173; D, 188; E, 50,
171, 173, 176, 179; E-2, 50, 173;
F, 100, 173, 175, 178, 188, 192;
G, 50, 173, 176, 179, 182, 183,
186, 190, 191
cataracts, 185-86
chalcone, 3
charcoal, powdered, 90
chelated minerals, 118, 149
chemical stress, 63
chemicalization of environment,
5, 16, 18, 20-21, 22
Chemistry in Therapeutics by
Walter B. Guy, M.D., 126
chicken pox, 102
Chico San products, 18, 19
chiropractic physicians, 10, 79
chlorophyll, 149
Chlorophyll Complex Perles, 179,
181, 184, 193
chlorine, 21
Cholacol II, 91, 147, 189

Choline, 147
citrinoids, 3
citrus, 3
Clark, Linda, 123, 126
clay, 91
clothes, dangerous chemicals in,
22
codeine, 92
coenzymes, 4
coffee, 2, 60, 155, 160, 162; enema,
92, 162
cold compresses, 98-99
cold feet, 87
colds, 75-76, 101-102, 121; vinegar
body rub for, 102
colitis, 38
Collinsonia root powder capsules,
95, 185
colonics, 10, 95
Comfrey-Pepsin capsules, 94, 150,
171, 189
compresses, vegetable, 104
constipation, 89-90, 164
Consumer Beware! by Beatrice
Trum Hunter, 126
contaminants, chemical, in processed foods, 6, 8, 16, 17, 96;
invading the body, 19-24; alimentary putrefactive, 52
coronary heart attacks, 27, 38
coronary occlusion, 100
corrective treatment in nutrition
therapy, 12
corticosteroids, 139
cortisone, 83, 84, 85, 86, 145
coughs, 102-103
cyanocobalamine, 146
cyclamates, 17, 120
cytotrophins, 10, 14, 23, 36, 47, 48,
149

d-alpha tocopherol, 88
Davis, Adelle, 122-23, 126
deceptive labeling, 15, 18-19
Denamone, 179
dentifrices, 21, 97-98
detoxification programs, 12, 13,
53, 54, 75, 80, 89, 147-48, 157,
159-60, 163-64, 168-69, functions
of liver in, 23
devitalized foods, 15

diabetes mellitus, 8, 38, 62, 64, 77-80, 137, 167, 181-82
diagnosis, 37-38, 43
diarrhea, 90-92
Diet and Disease by Emanuel Cheraskin et al., 126
diet, detoxifying, 10, 23, 44, 67, 69, 71, 82, 84, 86, 113, 139-40, 155, 166; raw food, 86; high protein, 94
dietetics, 113
diethylstilbesterol, 17
digestion, proper, 13, 51, 93, 138
digestive aids, 150
digitalis, 75
distribution of nutrients, 13
diversification of foods, need for, 3-4
dizziness, 67, 176-78
Doctor Who Looked at Hands, The, by John M. Ellis, M.D., 126
Drenaplex, 171, 189, 191
drugs, and drug-producing industry, 6, 13, 39, 44, 45, 81, 114, 116, 121, 139, 153, 157, 160
Dusty Miller plant, 106
dysinsulinism, 64, 79, 137
dysmenorrhea, 180-81

Ear, Nose and Throat Dysfunctions Due to Deficiencies and Imbalances by Sam E. Roberts, M.D., 127
ears, 158, 162, 167
eclectic physicians, 10
education in nutritional medicine, 24, 30, 31, 119-27 passim; of public, on hypoglycemia, 58-59
Eff-plus, 186, 187
electrocardiogram, 129, 159, 163, 168
electrolytes, 91
elimination, optimal, 13, 52, 138
emotional stress, 11, 63
endocrine glands, 64
enemas, 89, 95, 102, 162, 164; coffee, 92
enzymes, 4, 10, 12, 21, 48, 51, 95; pancreatic, 12, 51, 150
epsom salts, 92
ergosterol, 53

ethyl chloride, 100-101
Eustacian tube manipulation, 178
excretion, see elimination
exercise, 10; as preventive measure, 11; in corrective treatment, 12, 13; for prostate congestion, 99-100
Exhaustion: Causes and Treatment by Sam E. Roberts, M.D., 127
eyes, 158, 162, 167

fasting, 12, 95, 135; for diarrhea, 91
fats, 2, 7, 14, 82
fatty acids, 4
Feel Like a Million by Catharyn Elwood, 126
Ferroplus, 179, 185
fertilizers, natural, 18; synthetic, 5
fever, vinegar rub for relief of, 98
figs, black mission, 90, 95; compress of, 104
flax seed meal, 89
flea collars, 36
Fleet's Phosphosoda, 189
flora, beneficial intestinal, 91, 150; in mouth, 97
flue, 66, 68, 101-102
fluorides, 21
Food Facts and Fallacies by Dr. Carlton Fredericks and Herbert Bailey, 126
Food and Drug Administration (FDA), 24, 25
foods, whole natural and organic, 3, 4, 18-19, 46-47, 66; processed, 3, 6, 81, 121, 155; adulterated, 14, 20; synthetic, 16; raw, 47, 86
Fredericks, Dr. Carlton, 123-24
freezing, effect of, in food processing, 3

gallbladder colic, 92, 100
gallstones, 40, 92
garlic bud, peeled, as suppository, 95
garlic compress, 104
gas leaks, 19

gastrointestinal tract, contaminants in, 20-21
Get Well Naturally by Linda Clark, 126
gland extracts, 48, 50, 57. See also cytotrophins
glandular substances, desiccated, 13-14
glucose, intravenous, 139
glucose tolerance test, 56, 58, 64, 68, 128, 135-36, 159, 163, 168; criteria of interpretation of, 136-37; dynamics of, 138
glycerine, 90, 103
gynecologists, 67

hair, mineral evaluation test of, 130-31
Harris, Seale, M.D., 57, 139
hay fever, 158, 162
headaches, 66, 67, 85, 165, 166, 182-83
health food stores, 120
health foods, see foods, whole natural and organic
heart problems, 8, 50, 52, 72-75, 87-89, 100, 113, 158, 159, 163, 167, 172-73
heart tests, 129
heartburn, 93
heartogram, 2
heat, effect of, in food processing, 3, 16, 47
hemorrhoids, 94-96
Hepatrophin, 147, 189, 191
herbs, 10, 12, 18, 25, 44, 121
hereditary factors in health deterioration, 6
high blood pressure, 88
hives, allergic, nutritional aid in, 83-84
Hoffer-Osmond Diagnostic Test (HOD), 135, 159, 163, 168
homeopathic medicine, 10, 106
hormones, 88, 145; in foods, 16-17; therapy, sensitivity to, 82; assimilation, 82
hot compresses, 98-99
hydrochloric acid, 12, 51, 91, 96, 150; dilute, 146
hyperinsulinism, 61, 62, 63

hypertension, 113
hypoglycemia, 38, 79, 81, 83, 111, 155, 165; description and history of, 55-59; symptoms of, 59-61, 65, 66, 67-68, 160-61, 166; defined, 61; theory of, 61-62; misdiagnosis of, 61, 64; case histories of, 65-69; diagnosing, 128-38; treating, 138-50
Hypoglycemia Foundation, 56
hypoglycemic agent for diabetes control, 78, 79, 81
hysperidine, 3

injections, nutritional, 66, 79, 86, 138, 139, 159, 164, 168
Inositol, 182
insect repellant, 20
insecticides, see chemicalization of environment and pesticides
insomnia, 68, 160, 161, 190-92
insulin, 61-63
intake of nutrients, adequate, 51, 138
intestinal parasites, 94, 95-96
iodine, 102
Iodomere tablets, 102
iron, inorganic, 88

Journal International Academy of Applied Nutrition, 124
juices, 102

Kaopectate, 91
kelp, 102, 149
kidney problems, 166
kidney stones, 69-70
knee jerks, 163

lack of energy, 160, 161
lactic acidophilus yeast, 188, 189
laxatives, 164; natural, 89-90, 164
lecithin, 101-102; soy bean, 176
Lee, Dr. Royal, D.D.S., 118
Let's Eat Right to Keep Fit by Adelle Davis, 126
Let's Get Well by Adelle Davis, 126
Let's Have Healthy Children by Adelle Davis, 126
Let's Live Magazine, 41, 55, 125
licorice root tea, 191

liver extracts, 23, 48
liver function, 13, 22-23, 48, 62, 64, 92, 95, 138, 147. *See also* detoxification programs
low blood sugar, *see* hypoglycemia
Low Blood Sugar and You by Dr. Carlton Fredericks and Herman Goodman, 126
Low Fat Way to Health and Longer Life, The, by Lester M. Morrison, M.D., 127
lungs, 158, 163, 167; contaminants in, 19-20
lupus erythematosus, 80, 84-86
lysine, 3

magnesium oxide tablets, 70
magnesium sulfate, 149
malnutrition, 38, 43, 119, 140, 152, 159; as cause of disease, 44
margarine, 16
Matter of Life, A, by W. Coda Martin, M.D., 126
measles, 102
Medical World, 127
megacolon, 188-89
melon compress, 104
memory, poor, 87
menstruation, problems of, 164-65, 178-81
mental depression, 189-90
Metabolic Nutrition, 44. *See also* nutritional therapy
metabolism, normal, 13, 138; body-building factors in, 4; corrections in, 53
milk, simmered skim, 91
Miller Message, The, 125
Minaplex, 175, 182, 187, 191
minerals, 4, 7, 8, 10, 36, 44, 46, 47, 48, 91, 147-48, 159; trace, 97, 98, 173; chelated, 118, 149
Min Tran, 190
misdiagnosis of hypoglycemia, 61, 64; of heart problems, 100
mononucleosis, infectious, 158
Moor's tooth powder, 98
morphine, 92
mouth, 158, 162, 167
mouth therapy, 99

mouth washes, 21
mumps encephalitis, 162
Muncie technique (of Dr. Douglas Muncie), 178
mung bean sprouts, 96
My Battle with Low Blood Sugar by C.M. Thienell, 127

nasal congestion, 103
Natural Food and Farming, 125
natural foods, *see* foods, whole natural and organic
Natural Foods Cook Book, The, by Beatrice Trum Hunter, 126
natural remedies, 116
Nature Brand, Inc., 154
naturopathic physicians, 10
Neurotrophin, 177, 183
New Hope For Incurable Diseases by Emanuel Cheraskin *et al.,* 126
Niacinamide-B-6, 178, 185, 190
Nia-Plus, 190
nicotine, 19-20
Noxzema, 96
Nucleo-protein, 193
nutrient intake, proper, 13
nutrients, synthetic, 15
nutrition, defined, 1, 7-8; and body needs, 2-4; corrective, 12; therapy with, 12-14 *ff.*
Nutrition Abstracts & Reviews, 124
Nutrition and Health by Sir Robert McCarrison, M.D., and H.M. Sinclair, M.D., 126
Nutrition and Physical Degeneration by Weston A. Price, 127
Nutrition Today, 124
nutritional concept, basic, 18
nutritional research, 41-42, 115, 116, 123-24
nutritional stress, 63
nutritional therapy, 4, 30-31, 65, 111, 152-53; adverse body reactions to, 53-54
obesity, 113, 157, 158
ocean, harvesting food from, 5
Oculotrophin, 186
olive oil, 90
onion compress, 104

Orchex, 183, 190, 191
Organic Iodine, 189
organic nature of foods, guarantee
   of, 17-18
Organicville Newsletter, 125
osteopathic physicians, 10
Ostogen, 175, 187
Ovatrophin, 179, 180
Overfed but Undernourished by
   H. Curtis Wood, Jr., M.D., 127

pancreas, 61-62, 63, 64; enzymes
   of, 12, 51, 150
Pancreatrophin, 182
Pap smear, 159, 168
papaya compress, 104
papaya tooth powder, 98
paralysis, 29
Parotid Cytotrophin, 181
Pauling, Dr. Linus, 121
pellagra, 157
pelvic examination, 158, 167-68
penicillin, 45
pepsin, 12, 51, 150
periodicals containing nutrition
   information, 24-25
pesticides, 5, 16, 21, 119
phenacetin, 92
phonocardiogram, 2, 129
Phosphade, 173, 176, 178, 183,
   186
photographs, diagnostic evaluation by means of, 135, 150
physical deterioration, causes of,
   6-7
physical stress, 63
physiotherapy, 12, 13
pill, contraceptive, 71, 121, 167
pineapple compress, 104
pituitary gland, 64
Pituitrophin, 180, 182, 183, 186
Pneumatrophin, 171
poison oak and ivy, 106
pollution, food, 5
population explosion, 5
potato, raw, as suppository, 95;
   compress of grated, 104
prednisone, 80, 81
pregnancy, nutritional aid, in,
   71-72
pregnancy schedule, 183-85

preservatives, 14-15, 16, 21
pressure spray containers, 19
Prevention magazine, 19, 125
preventive measures in nutrition
   therapy, 11, 37-39
processed foods, 3, 6, 81, 121, 155
prostate congestion, 99-100
Prostate Cytotrophin tablets, 100,
   192
prostatic hypertrophy, benign,
   192-93
Prostex, 183, 186, 187
proteins, 2, 7, 14; powders, milk,
   94
protein bound iodine test, 128
protomorphogens, 12, 14, 23, 47-
   48, 149
Protomorphology by Royal Lee,
   D.D.S., and William A. Hanson,
   126
psoriasis, 175-76
pulse, 158, 162, 167
pulsogram, 129, 159, 163, 168
pyridoxine, 146

quality of products, 153-54
quercitin, 3
Quinidine, 78

radish sprouts, 96
raisins, 90
raw food, 47; diet, 86
rectal itching, 95
recycling of nitrogenous wastes,
   24-25
Renatrophin, 185
Rhus Tox, 106
riboflavin, 47
Ribo-Nucleic Acid, 193
Rodale's Health Bulletin, 125
Rogoff's sign, 163
Rutaplex, 186
Ruta-Plus, 183
rutin, 3

saccharine, 17
salt, 2, 56; solar dried sea or earth,
   89, 91, 95, 97, 105, 178
salt water, 104, 105
Science, 124
scurvy, 39, 43

sea water, 106
Secrets of Health and Beauty by Linda Clark, 126
seed sprouts, 25
seeds, nutritional importance of, 18
Selye, Hans, M.D., 11, 57, 63, 139
senna leaves, powdered, 90
Seromins, 178, 181
Seroyd Brands, Inc., 154
shingles, 102
shortenings, nonfood, 16
shortness of breath, 88
Shute, Evan, M.D., 89
Shute, Wilfred E., 88-89
skin and skin problems, 104, 158, 159, 162, 167, 175-76; contaminants in, 21-22; nutritional aid for, 80-81
slippery elm bark, powdered, 90
smog, 19
smoking, 19-20, 60
soaps, dangers of, 21-22
soda, bicarbonate of, 97
sodium chloride, 149
sodium propionate, 15
soft drinks, 15
sore throat, 43
soured milk, 45
Soy Bean Lecithin, 176
sponge tablets, 102
sprays, chemical, 18, 19; residue on produce, 96
sprouted seeds, 96-97
squash seeds, 100
Standard Process Laboratories, 118, 154
starches, natural, 4, 61
Stay Young Longer by Linda Clark, 123, 126
stress, types of, 63
stress-adaptation syndrome, 57, 58, 61, 63
stroke, 77-80
Studies in Deficiency Disease by Sir Robert McCarrison, M.D., 126
sugar, 2, 4, 86, 138-39
Summary, The, 125
sun, exposure to, for treating poison oak and ivy, 106

Sun Circle products, 17, 20
Sun Valley products, 18, 19, 154
supplements, natural nutritional, 11, 12, 13, 18, 28, 36, 46, 66, 71, 86, 117, 139, 147-50
suppositories, 95
sweeteners in foods, 17
sweets, 60, 62, 174. See also sugar
surgery, 6, 12, 13, 14, 39, 40, 94, 139; open-heart, 74
synergistic factors in vitamins, 3

Target Diet, 140
Taub, Harold, 88-89
temperature, 158, 162, 167
tension, 11
therapeutic measures in nutritional practice, 12-14
therapeutic programs outlined, 159-60, 163-64, 168-69
thought patterns, body functions and, 11
Thymex, 176
Thymus, 172
Thytrophin, 179, 186, 188, 189, 193
tin can linings, danger of, 16
Tintera, John, M.D., 57, 63, 139
tocopherols, 88
tonsillectomies, 40
toothbrushing, 21, 97-98
trace minerals, 37, 97, 98, 173, 186
tranquilizers, 68, 139
Trapper's Ointment, 104

ulcer syndrome, nutritional aid for, 81-82
ulcers, 38, 43, 93-94, 113
urine tests, 85, 129, 130, 159, 163, 168
USF (unsaturated fatty acid ointment), 159
Utrophin, 179

vacuum dehydration of foods, 18, 25, 118
vaginitis, 165, 166
vinegar, apple cider, 91, 93, 96, 98, 102, 106, 149; wine, 93
Viobin Corp., 154
vitamin complexes, explanation of, 3

Vitamin E for Ailing and Healthy Hearts by Wilfrid E. Shute and Harold J. Taub, 127

Vitamin E: Your Key to a Healthy Heart by Herbert Bailey, 126

Vitamin Products Company, 118, 154

vitamins, 4, 10, 36, 44, 46, 47, 48-49, 79, 84, 91, 147, 159, 166; B_{12}, 27, 29, 47, 48, 146; B_2, 47; B_{22}, 48; B_6, 126, 146; with niacinamide, 178, 185, 190; C, 3 20, 43, 47, 94, 102, 105, 115, 121, 146, 175, 176, 180; D, synthetic, 53; E, 49, 50, 87-89, 105-6, 115; F, 106; K, 3; A & C (urea), 172, 191; B Supreme, 190

vitamins, synthetic, 13, 27, 48-49, 53

Vitamins in Medicine, The, by Franklin Bicknell, M.D., and Frederick Prescott, M.D., 126

warts, 106-7

water, 4, 7, 102; chlorinated, danger of, 21; warm salt, for constipation, 89

Westpro Laboratories, 154

wheat germ oil perles, 171, 173

wheat seed sprouts, 96

Williams, Dr. Roger I., 123-24

X-ray, 14

yogurt, 45

You Are Extraordinary by Roger J. Williams, 127

Zymex II capsules, 95, 172

Zypan, 175, 176